Success Is Just Running Out of Mistakes:

A Lifelong Quest to Make Hemodialysis

Simple, Safe, and Effective

by

Stephen R. Ash, MD, FACP

*The two most important days in your
life are the day you are born
and the day you find out
why.*
—Mark Twain

Table of Contents

Introduction

I remember the first time I saw a hemodialysis machine in operation, on a patient with acute renal failure. It was in 1970 on the second floor of the University of Kansas Medical Center in Kansas City, where I was a third-year medical student. It was an RSP machine with a 100-liter tank of dialysate, twin-coil kidney, and the access was two single-lumen catheters, one in the femoral artery and the other in the femoral vein. I was amazed by two things. First was how remarkable it was that the function of the human kidney, so selective in determining excretion of thousands of various metabolites and toxins, could be somehow replicated by a collection of cellophane membranes and salt water. Second was how beautifully simple but how crude the machine was. A roller pump propelled blood through a collection of tubing's, then through a dialyzer with cellulosic membranes and returned it to the blood. Pressure in the circuit was monitored by a mercury switch. I had seen more sophisticated technology in the 1931 Buick Business Coupe that I drove in high school.

By that time, I was already fascinated by the kidney, with its complex interplay of so many tissues in providing so many functions to the body. Especially I was amazed by its regenerative capacity. Dr. Jared Grantham had shown me how to dissect living kidney tubules and how to measure their function in vitro. Each summer of my first two years I worked in the pathology laboratories, and I wrote my first scientific article on the metabolic changes that occur when the kidney decides to regenerate.

For Internship, Residency and Fellowship I went to Indiana University Medical School, mostly because my young wife Marianne wished to be closer to her home. My training at IUMC was a great experience, tiring, but great. When I had the chance to do research in my third year of Residency I studied the origin of cells which regenerate kidneys, and tried to grow tubule cells on artificial membranes. However, by then I already realized that hemodialysis was going to be very impractical as a long-term therapy for End Stage Renal Disease (ESRD). There had to be a better answer. There were dramatic improvements in hemodialysis going on at the time of my fellowship, and I was thankful for seeing them first at IUMC: hollow fiber dialyzers, controlled filtration, proportioning machines and bicarbonate dialysate. But none of these made dialysis simpler. I began to read literature related to artificial kidneys and see what alternatives were available. I was captivated by the development of the Redy™ machine and the Sorb™ column. Not only were many of the numerous uremic toxins able to pass through a dialyzer membrane, but every toxin we knew about was bound by a column containing four layers, and three of them inorganic: charcoal, urease, zirconium phosphate cation exchanger and zirconium oxide anion exchanger. I also read the proceedings of the yearly NIH Contractors conferences and learned of other approaches for removal of uremic toxins from dialysate, and a number of ideas for oral sorbents. Perhaps it was my undergrad degree in Physics that made me continue to look for the simplest possible solutions.

At the conclusion of Fellowship in Nephrology, I traveled to the University of Utah to work for three months in the Department of Nephrology but also in the Artificial Organs Division, with Dr. Willlem Kolff, who was developing the Wearable Artificial Kidney (WAK). On returning to Lafayette, Indiana I joined the Arnett Clinic (a multispecialty group) and opened the Hemodialysis Laboratory within the newly formed Bioengineering Department at Purdue University. That was in 1975, and still today my research focuses on making dialysis simple, safe, and suited for the home environment. The research continued from the Bioengineering Department into private companies formed by me and my business partner, Mr. Bob Truitt. Each company has its own interesting story of the pathway to success or failure with the projects. This document is a biography, not just of people, but of companies and of ideas. It is apparent that dialysis therapy began to stabilize (or crystallize) in the last few decades, while it was expanding greatly in the "in-center dialysis unit" business model. Many articles have been written about the "lack of innovation" in Nephrology, and questioned why it is that there are no new ideas or devices in dialysis therapy. One reason I wrote this biography is to demonstrate that there has been no dearth of new ideas in dialysis therapy. If as a single practicing physician, I can find and develop twelve new technologies to MAYBE answer major problems in therapy of ESRD, then certainly any nephrologist in practice could do the same. Maybe not twelve times, but at least a few times. The main problem has been that even when many of the new approaches were shown to be safe and effective alternatives to standard practice of dialysis, the was a lack of desire for real change on the part of most nephrologists. To be early adopters of new technology requires a lot of work and effort, real curiosity and a dose of courage. The major dialysis equipment manufacturers found that most nephrologists wanted evolutionary, not revolutionary changes in hemodialysis machinery. It's maybe too harsh to say "no one cared" because some of our projects were wildly successful and well accepted by the market. But for most of them, the statement is close to true. As Pogo said in the famous comic strip, "We have met the enemy and it is us."

There are twelve chapters in this biography. Each represents a separate project I worked on during my career. All of these projects had the general goal of making hemodialysis simpler, safer and more suited for use in the home. Table 1 gives a synopsis of each project, the location of work, the product and the eventual out-come. **Figure 1** includes a listing of the numerous steps which are necessary to carry an idea for a new product to market introduction. The vertical lines show the course of each of the twelve projects, and indicate the step at which many of the projects failed. Out of twelve projects and products, only two at this time have entered widespread clinical use and become a market success in the U.S. The biography therefore should be somewhat of a warning for physicians, scientists and engineers who are also inventors and entrepreneurs and decide to develop a new device or drug. This is an exciting and worthy endeavor. However, the road to market success is long, and even after FDA approval of your new product, there are many potholes and barriers. To help you out, at the end of each chapter I reflect on the lessons we learned in the course of the project, and what contributed to success or failure of the project. To the credit of my colleagues in our research projects, we generally only made each mistake once. And perhaps, success is just being so persistent that you just run out of mistakes before you run out of miracles.

At the request of Dr. Paul Malchesky (past editor of Artificial Organs), and Dr. Vakhtang Tchantchaleishvili (present editor), I have published much of this book in the journal during 2022. Artificial Organs has a long history of publishing histories which describe important people and events in the history of artificial organs, and I feel honored by their invitation to share my experiences (good and bad) in attempting to improve dialysis therapy. The Introduction was published in January, 2022 and chapters were published, one each month, during the entire year[1].

Year	Location	Project	Clinical Trials.	FDA Approval	Outcome
1975	Artificial Organs Dept, U. of Utah	1.WAK: Invented by Dr. Kolff and Dr. Jacobsen, a single access machine with charcoal regeneration of dialysate, plus small dialysate tank for removal of small m.w. toxins.	Yes	N/A	Successful device, licensee decided to make it more complete, but not "wearable." Device never marketed.
1975-1983	Bioengineering Center, Purdue Univ.	2.SSRD: Wearable HD system using sorbent suspension and reciprocating membranes to pump blood through single access. Cooperation with Union Carbide in developing calcium-loaded zeolites for binding potassium and ammonium+ from urea.	No	No	Ca- loaded zeolites worked perfectly but released aluminum and/or silica to dialysate. Project funding cancelled by major company.
1983-1988	Ash Medical Systems	3.BioLogic-HD™ with dialysate regeneration (Redy™), single access, plate dialyzer membranes as blood pump, airless blood circuit, controlled filtration and automatic fluid replacement.	No	1986	Worked well physically, some technical problems that were resolvable. CMS cancelled home helpers in 1986 and home dialysis market evaporated in 1987. Venture capital companies "walked."
1989-1997	HemoCleanse	4.BioLogic-DT™ similar to BioLogic-HD but with liter sorbent suspension. Indications: hepatic encephalopathy and drug overdose.	Yes	1997	Licensed to spin-off company HemoTherapies, marketed therapy as Liver Dialysis. They failed to focus on A-on-C hepatic failure, and on the large liver transplant centers as planned. Clinical results were variable. Licensee went bankrupt.

Table 1: Twelve projects aimed at making hemodialysis simple, safe, and effective in the home environment (Ash and many collaborators)

2000 2007	HemoCleanse and spin-off Renal Solutions	5. Allient™ HD machine with hollow-fiber dialyzer, single- or dual-access, pressure actuated blood pumping, dialysate regeneration (Redy™), controlled filtration and automatic fluid replacement	Yes	2006	Company (including Sorb, Inc.) sold to FMC in 2007. Plan was to redesign machine but this never happened and project eventually was cancelled.
2002-2015	HemoCleanse and spin-off ZS Pharma	6. Zirconium cyclosilicate: After above project using zeolites, Union Carbide and UOP developed a crystal designed for binding monovalents like potassium and ammonium+. HemoCleanse performed early animal studies to test ZS as an oral sorbent and helped to form ZS Pharma as the sole licensee in 2008. HemoCleanse helped direct product development and plan clinical trials.	Yes	2018	ZS Pharma was sold to AstraZeneca in 2015. The highly successful oral powder for removing potassium is now on market as Lokelma. HemoCleanse retained rights to use of as extracorporeal sorbent.
1996-2000	Ash Access	7. Ash Split-Cath™ chronic central venous catheter (CVC) for hemodialysis	Yes	1997	Highly successful, first split-tip CVC for dialysis. Patent was more restrictive than needed, so competitive catheters appeared on the market. Royalty arrangement with MedComp ended with a buy-out.
1997-2000	Ash Access	8. Concentrated sodium citrate catheter lock: We showed the antibacterial and anticoagulant effects of concentrate sodium citrate in a published paper with clinical results in 2000. We stated that 47% concentration left catheters quickly due to density. The article recommended a concentration of 23% sodium citrate as catheter lock, made by diluting 47% sodium citrate (instructions for use repeated this direction).	Yes	N/A	US and PCT patents were issued. The patent was contested by a Netherlands company in PCT court and they won on appeal. After one accidental over-injection of the product, product, FDA issued a warning and limitations on product use in 2000. Remains on the market in Europe and worldwide today and its use has been shown to decrease CRBSI incidence.

Year	Location	Project	Clinical Trials	FDA Approval	Outcome
2004-2014	Ash Access	9. Zuragen®: A catheter lock at 7% concentration (for density equal to blood) and parabens and methylene blue to provide antibacterial function. Sponsored large randomized clinical trial to demonstrate safety and benefits.	Yes	No	FDA decided the product was a drug due to antibacterial functions. Clinical trial showed significant decrease in infections by concordant cultures, but lock not approved to market. Licensee abandoned project, product re-licensed.
2014-present	Ash Access and spin-off Zurex Pharma	10. Zuragard™:Skin preparation solution with components of Zuragen and 70% isopropyl alcohol. Zuragen catheter lock is a potential product also.	Yes	Yes	Zuragard has been shown in clinical trials to be more effective than Chloroprep® in decreasing skin bacteria. Beta site testing now being performed.
2014-present	Ash Access	11. 7% sodium citrate with benzyl alcohol: Concentration of sodium citrate the same as Zuragen® but added benzyl alcohol as preservative	Plann-ed	503B now reg. app. plann-ed	Now marketed through a compounding pharmacy. Clinical trial planned for general approval as a routine catheter lock for dialysis patients.
2010-present	HemoCleanse	12. Sterile carbon block/Oral Uremic Toxin Sorbent: Carbon block to remove middle molecule toxins from dialysate and mixed ion exchangers taken orally to remove small, charged uremic toxins.	Plann-ed	Plann-ed	Both projects are still in development and testing phases, carbon block is licensed,new oral sorbent under evaluation by a major drug company.

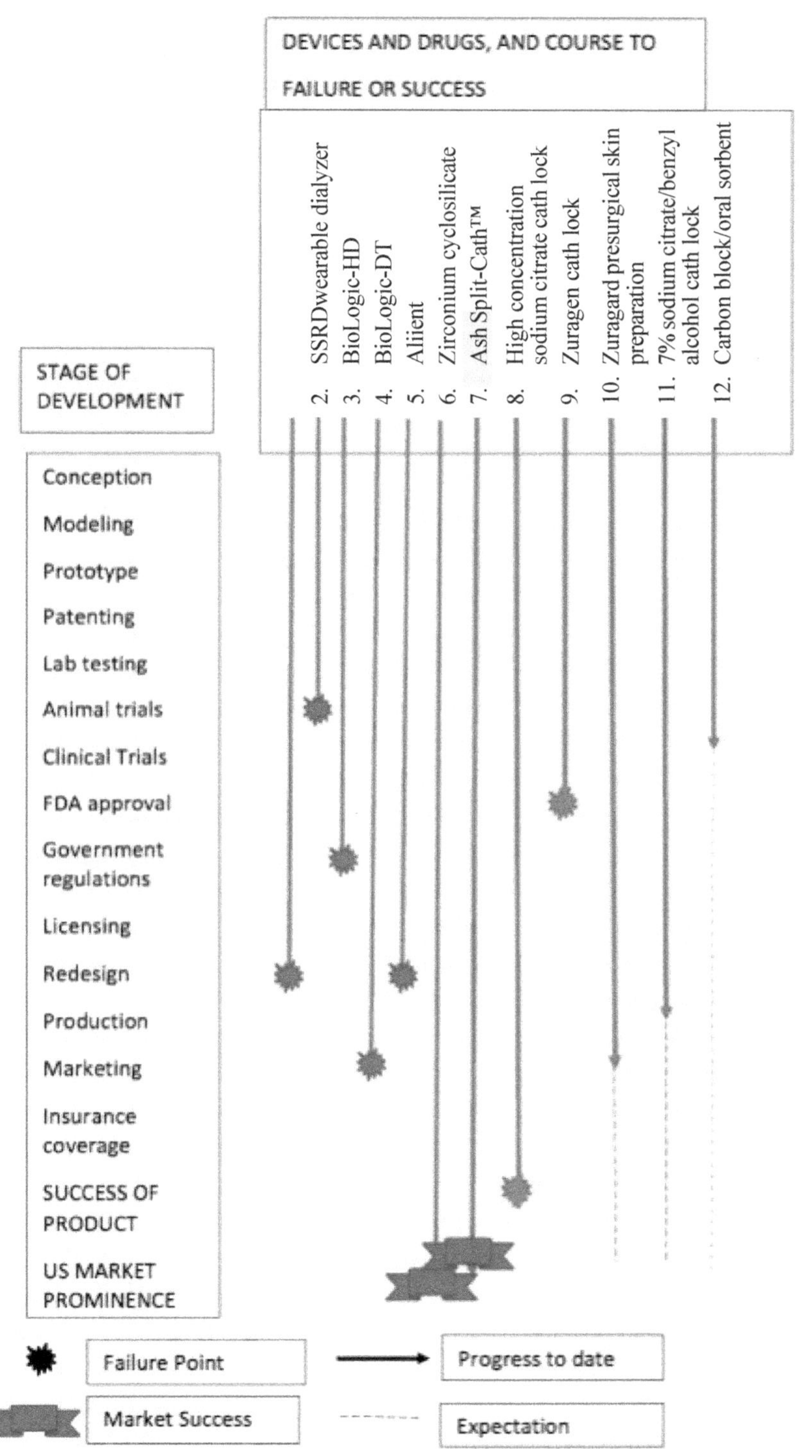

Figure 1. Progress of various research projects to make dialysis simple, safe and effective in the home environment. Note that project failures occurred at many of the steps from invention to widespread clinical use. *Blue lines:* sorbent-based dialysis and oral therapies. *Red lines:* catheters and catheter locks and pre-op skin preparation.

Chapter 1:

The Wearable Artificial Kidney
created by Kolff and Jacobsen

when I first read about the Wearable Artificial Kidney (WAK), invented by Dr. Willem Kolff and a mechanical engineer Dr. Stephen Jacobsen, I felt I just had to see this. Here was a battery-powered single access hemodialysis machine with sorbent regeneration of dialysate. [2], [3] How close was this to the market? How far had it been proven? What were the limitations? I arranged a three-month temporary appointment as Assistant Professor in the Nephrology department at the University of Utah in the summer of 1975. My appointment actually started in the last month of my Fellowship in Nephrology at Indiana University School of Medicine (were they being generous or did they want to get rid of this guy?). Dr. Kolff graciously accepted me into the Artificial Organs department and immediately gave me some assignments related to the WAK project.

The WAK (Figure 2) was a real device, with an ingenious design allowing single-needle dialysis (drawing blood out of a vein and returning it through the same single needle)[4]. It had an ingenious pump with a plate that alternately com- pressed tubing containing dialysate and blood and recovered energy normally lost in tubing com- pression[5]. This function automatically created back-and-forth filtration across the membranes,

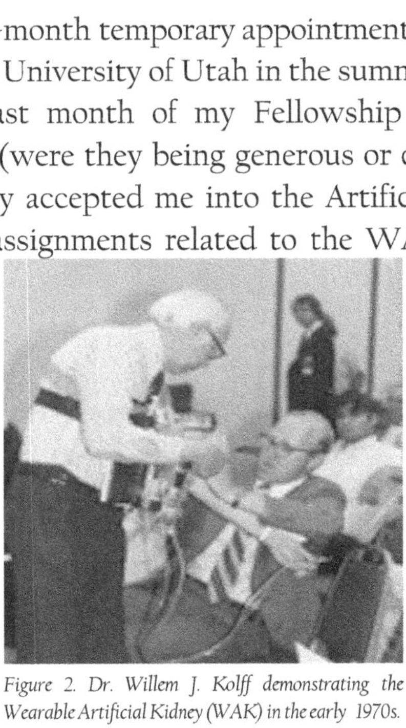

Figure 2. Dr. Willem J. Kolff demonstrating the Wearable Artificial Kidney (WAK) in the early 1970s.

which should increase removal of middle molecular weight toxins. To my surprise the WAK didn't include a complete sorbent column. The wearable part of the system had only a charcoal column for toxin removal, sufficient for removing organic toxins, but not the small and charged uremic toxins. For removal of phosphate, urea and potassium a twenty-liter tank with pre-heated dialysate was attached into the dialysate lines of the machine for ninety minutes during each daily treatment and then removed and replaced by a second tank. This was adequate for removal of the small and charged toxins and also for providing buffers to correct acidosis (lactate or acetate, back then). Patients tolerated the treatments well, and even took trips down the Colorado River while using the device.

The experience at the AO department of the University of Utah was amazing. Here were a number of skilled engineers involved in product development with a genius inventor and physician on a radical improvement in dialysis therapy for many ESRD patients. Dr. Jacobsen was also a remarkable engineer and inventor of numerous biomedical devices. Additionally, the Nephrology group (including Drs. Elizabeth Atkin-Thor and Dr. Robert Stephens) were innovative and introduced me to many new alternative technologies, including peritoneal dialysis for ESRD, peritoneal catheters, the Redy™ System with its sorbent column, AV shunts for blood access, and so on. My work and stay at the University of Utah was only for one summer. I loved the Artificial Organs department, Dr. Kolff, the University, and of course the remarkable land- scape of Utah. But my wife Marianne was in Veterinary School at Purdue University, and there was no Vet School in Salt Lake City. Further, we had just purchased an 1870 farm house in Lafayette, which needed a lot of work, and we had a three-year-old daughter Emily. So, I was bound to return to Lafayette. Also, I had my own ideas about how the wearable artificial kidney should work, so perhaps it was best if I set up my own laboratory to see if the ideas worked. While at the University of Utah I had been tasked with coming up with a new way to sterilize dialyzers between use, which was successful but not further pursued. I also devised a way to modify the WAK single-access blood path for use with an AV shunt. The greatest compliment I ever received was when, just before I left Salt Lake City, Dr. Kolff said "I underestimated you."

Over the years, I continued a long and supportive friendship with Dr. Kolff, as did most of his trainees. But the outcome of the WAK was disappointing. Dr. Jacobsen said a big problem was that after a major investment from an "Angel" investor, Kolff was in a hurry to bring the product to market, and there were some technical problems and deficiencies. The anti-recirculation valve for the single access system sometimes failed. Monitors in the device were minimal, for example there were no pressure monitors included on the blood or dialysate side. Dr. Jacobsen never had a chance to re-design or improve the product.

I contributed only a little to the WAK project, and in fact when I asked Kolff why he didn't just use a Redy™ (Sorb™) column to regenerate dialysate he said "It's too heavy and too complicated."[6] I felt that a sorbent column for all uremic tox- ins was necessary for the device to be complete. Years later and after much experience I had to admit that he was right about the sorbent column. There were many technical problems in the use of the Sorb™ column that our team encountered when we actually built it into a sophisticated dialysis machine: excess removal of calcium and magnesium, sodium release, acid release, high perfusion pressure, and varying fluid volume in the column to mention a few (see Chapters 3 and 5).

Kolff licensed the WAK to a Japanese company that liked the overall features, but when they designed the product to fit the market they saw, it was no longer portable and not sorbent based. A traditional proportioning dialysate delivery system was built into the machine. As shown in **Figure 1 and Table 1** of the Introduction I think the main failure of the WAK project was in the re-design phase. Re-design for production occurs whenever a prototype is licensed to an existing company making medical equipment. In the process of in the process of re-design, the WAK lost its portability and its ability to use minimal volumes of water. It became a stationary dialysis system with excellent removal of uremic toxins (especially if used daily) and a great advantage of providing single-needle access. But single-needle dialysis means that the outflow of blood through the needle is interrupted during return of blood. This means that the blood treatment rate is about half of that for standard dual-needle dialysis and the clearances, especially for small toxins like urea decrease proportionally. Extending the duration of dialysis will make up for lower clearance rates, but this is really practical only in the home setting. By the late 1970s the mania in the US was for faster and faster in-center dialysis, not slow home hemodialysis. Home hemodialysis was almost non-existent in Japan, so the company redesigned the product for the market that they perceived, foregoing the possibility of wearability or even portability.

LESSONS LEARNED:
    A. Be highly cautious in answering the question "when will this therapy be on the market to help patients?" Make sure that you know who will produce it and the production schedule before giving a firm date to an investor or pa- tient or collaborator.

B. For a therapy like dialysis which has predictable results, make the device as complete as possible before clinical trials. Optimize the device, include all needed components and monitors, and define the best user response to any problems that can be envisioned.

C. Have a balance of R&D in the team. If there's a component which is really needed but not available or unsuitable (such as a sorbent column), plan a long-term research program to create this component. That project will continue no matter what happens to the
original device.

D. Find a corporate partner with marketing plans which match with your device's potential.

E. Find a corporate partner with marketing plans which match with your de- vice's potential. Most large companies prefer to license and manufacture products which are evolutionary rather than revolutionary. That's what has made them large and successful.

F. Realize that new ideas and inventions have a life of their own, and they speak louder than words or pictures. Their very creation shows a need in the market and a frustration with the current technology and they demonstrate how to use other technology in a new approach. The WAK embodied Dr. Kolff's dream of a wearable kidney but it would also have been very successful as a very portable home dialysis machine. The WAK was never commercialized. However, four decades later, we still see the need for a dialysis system with single needle blood access, sorbent for removing toxins from dialysate, and high portability. This would make home dialysis simpler, safer and more efficient, just as Kolff envisioned. [7]

Chapter 2

The Sorbent Suspension Reciprocating Dialyzer; a Wearable Artificial Kidney that Almost Was

In order to pursue the dream of a wearable artificial kidney I visited Purdue University Bioengineering Department, which had just formed in 1975. The new director was soon to be Dr. Les Geddes, well-known for his work in cardiac electrophysiology at Baylor. Dr. Charlie Babbs convinced Dr. Geddes that having me in the department would be "like having a whole different Panzer division." Meanwhile, I joined a multi-specialty group called Arnett Clinic as their first Nephrologist. Since they didn't really know what a Nephrologist did, I thought I would have some extra time on my hands, so I made them a deal; I would spend every morning in clinical practice and every afternoon in the research lab, pursuing new devices and therapies. They said "Okay." So all-of-a-sudden I was in charge of the "Hemodialysis Laboratory" at the Bioengineering Center of Purdue University.

Our first project was to develop a truly simple, portable, and wearable hemodialysis system. I thought of every possible way to remove uremic toxins from blood with the minimum of mechanical and blood-contacting components. So, the Sorbent Suspension Reciprocating Dialyzer (SSRD) was born[8,9]. The idea was to use the

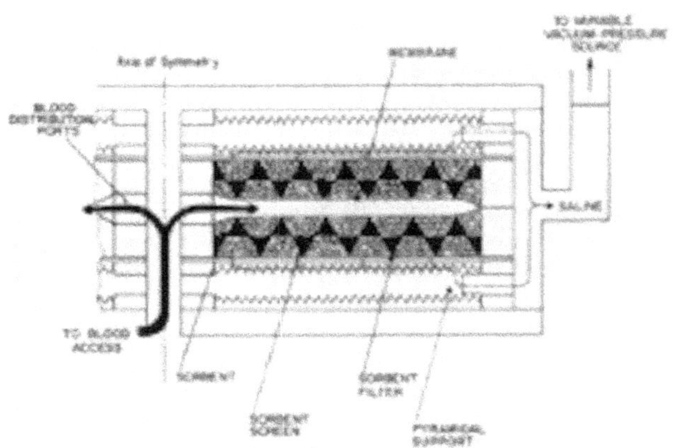

Figure 3. The SSRD, shown during blood inflow. Negative pressure ex- pands plate membranes to draw in blood and mix sorbent suspension next to the flat plate membranes. Positive pressure reverses blood and sorbent suspension flow.

membranes of a circular flat plate dialyzer to draw blood from a vein by applying vacuum to expand them, and return the blood by applying positive pressure to the membranes (Figure 3). A suspension of powdered sorbents on the outside of the membranes would act as a continuous "chemical sink" for removal of these toxins This was simplest de- sign possible for a wearable artificial kidney.

Somewhat miraculously, due to the way that sheet cellophane expands in one direction and contracts in another when it is wet, little folds developed in the Cuprophane® membranes. If the folds of each sheet were placed perpendicular to the other sheet, channels were formed so that the membranes emptied completely during each cycle. Similar to the rotating drum kidney, the membranes came to apposition after passing each bolus of blood, which removed layers of stagnant blood from the surface of the membranes[10]. This complete emptying was helpful in mass transfer because it eliminated all the stagnant blood layers that develop with flow-through dialyzer systems. It also meant a shortened residence time for the blood within the membranes, which should minimize clotting of blood in the system.

In the SSRD we used screen membrane supports, so the layers of blood attained a uniform thickness at full expansion. Applying pressure and vacuum to the fluid outside of the membranes not only propelled the blood into and out of the membranes but effectively mixed and replenished sorbent suspension at the membrane surface. The mixing of the sorbent side was demonstrated by maintenance of the removal rates of transfer of creatinine from a simulated blood solution into a powdered charcoal suspension, as confirmed by Dr. Linda Wang in our laboratory. The same was true for other organic compounds such as drugs[9]. Ultrafiltration rate was controlled by varying the time of delay after filling the packages, before starting outflow. Everything about the SSRD worked even better than we expected.

We knew that the dialyzer market was moving towards use of hollow fiber mem- branes rather than flat plate membranes. We tried repeatedly to find ways to mix a suspension of powdered sorbents around hollow fiber dialyzer membranes, using all kinds of agitation, pressure changes and even ultrasound energy to mix the sorbents. The layer of charcoal right next to the membrane remained stationary, as shown by the rapid diminution in efficiency of removal of organic toxins from the blood side. Also, plate membranes had biocompatibility advantage over hollow fibers, partly due to the fact that smooth gaskets distributed the blood flow from the inlet port instead of the somewhat jagged cut ends of the fibers and potting materials. So, we decided to stay with plate membranes in the SSRD.

All that we needed to do next was to devise a sorbent suspension that would re- move all of the uremic toxins from blood. Powdered activated charcoal was one essential element, for binding organic toxins. Urease could rapidly split urea in the dialysate. But if zirconium phosphate were used to remove ammonium and potassium, then calcium and magnesium would be removed from the blood and a re-in- fusion of calcium into the blood would be needed, as it is for dialysate in the Redy® system. Also, zirconium phosphate ion exchange compounds were so dense that they couldn't be made into a stable suspension. I decided to make a few presentations to Purdue University departments, asking if there isn't a cation ex- changer that is selective for monovalent cations over divalent cations, and maybe one with a lower density. At Chemical Engineering I was told that I should contact Dr. Joe White in Agronomy. Ion exchange is a large part of the function of soil. So, I made a presentation at the Ag School, and met Dr. Joe White. He was working with Dr. John Sherman of Union Carbide to develop and test synthetic zeolites (aluminosilicate crystals) for binding ammonium in the soil and in the guts of ruminants. Some versions of zeolites had been created which could be loaded with calcium and exchange the calcium for ammonium or potassium[11]. Bingo! We had Dr. Sherman come to Lafayette and give a presentation to my small research group. It was during that presentation that I realized that the calcium released during this exchange would bind phosphate and therefore avoid need for an anion exchanger in the sorbent sus- pension, control the sorbent suspension pH, and return about the right amount of bicarbonate to the patient. There would be no need for infusion of calcium and magnesium to the dialysate. We went forward full speed in collaboration with Union Carbide and soon had healthy support for the SSRD from the Eli Lilly company, since they were then involved in a number of device markets including peritoneal dialysis (through subsidiary Physio Control) in the late 1970s. Companies already in the hemodialysis market were not interested in radically simpler dialysis therapies, and felt the concept of a "wearable artificial kidney" was "far out."

The development of the SSRD went well. Eli Lilly contributed a covalently bound urease in the sorbent and offered their animal testing facilities for further tests. Union Carbide worked tirelessly on a series of synthetic zeolites with varying binding and affinity for calcium, ammonium, and potassium. During benchtop and animal tests, the blood chemistry changes created by the device were perfect and there was safety of operation, The SSRD worked exceedingly well.

We then performed toxicology studies during dialysis of normal animals. We discovered that the synthetic zeolites were solubilizing and releasing aluminum into dialysate, and this crossed the membrane into the blood. In vitro studies had not shown such solubility of the zeolites, but there were some dialyzable chemicals in blood that apparently increased the solubility of zeolites. The simple solution was to add silica to the zeolite suspension to bind the free aluminum. However, the next animal studies showed that the SSRD transferred enough silica across the dialyzer membranes to cause renal insufficiency in animals. This was totally unexpected. The common wisdom was that silica in blood was unrelated to any toxicity, and renal disease due to soluble silica in the blood had never been reported before. However, no one had made a dialysis system with a sorbent suspension partly made of zeolites.

We discussed various technical solutions to the problem of aluminum and silica re-lease from the zeolites (such as micro-encapsulation). But then there was a totally unexpected setback to Eli Lilly. The new NSAID Oraflex was shown to have toxicities in market populations at a greater rate than in clinical trials, and Eli Lilly withdrew Oraflex from the market. With the loss of the profitability from Oraflex, Eli Lilly cancelled all extra-mural research projects in cost-saving efforts. We were one of them. With the news that funding by Eli Lilly would cease soon, I announced to my assembled R&D team that the Hemo Dialysis laboratory at the Bioengineering department would be closing.

The future of our research team looked pretty bleak, but with the help of a skilled local businessman and scientist Mr. Bob Truitt, we soon formed a privately-held company named "Ash Medical" to pursue a sorbent-based dialysis system for treatment of kidney failure in the home. The plan was to capture many of the benefits of the SSRD in a system with a commercial plate dialyzer and Sorb™ sorbent column. But as a second application, could we use the same system with a sorbent suspension, in treatment of drug over dose and liver failure? When I was at the University of Utah, I had made one of the daily "morning presentations" to the Artificial Organ department and Dr. Kolff, and described my plans for something like the SSRD. At the end of the presentation, Kolff's response was "you need to learn about bird lungs." I didn't know why he made the comment but I read about bird lungs. Bird lungs have unidirectional airflow through "parabronchi" and cross-flow of blood in capillaries, and as they expand and contract, they propel air unidirectionally through the lungs. What Kolff meant (I think) was that we could use a standard flat plate dialyzer with screen supports in our sorbent suspension system and use the membrane to pump blood in and out of a single-access We tested such an application using a sorbent suspension on the dialysate side of a Cobe screen-plate dialyzer at the Hemo Dialysis lab in the last months it was open. It worked superbly, so we then had a general concept for a machine to treat kidney failure and which could then be adapted to treat drug overdose and liver failure.

So, with Bob, we launched Ash Medical. The dialysis machine project became more feasible and affordable when we used commercially available plate dialyzers and didn't have to make our own dialyzers. Ash Medical used the concepts to pro- duce the BioLogic-HD™ and BioLogic-DT™ systems, as described in later chapters. Some years later, at an ASAIO meeting I met Dr. Kolff and asked him if he remembered making the comment to me about bird's lungs. He said didn't remember it, but I certainly did.

LESSONS LEARNED:
    A. Don't rely on common knowledge when venturing into uncommon territory, such as placing aluminosilicate cation exchangers into dialysate.
    B. Don't proceed to animal trials of a device before investigating every possible problem of the components, in our case by seeing whether any of the chemicals in plasma made zeolites more soluble.
    C. Realize that when a product is revolutionary, rather than evolutionary, it is unlikely to interest companies already established in a medical market.
    D. When you have single-source funding for a large project it can disappear for reasons totally out of your control.
    E. Always have a back-up plan.

Chapter 3
BioLogic-HD™ and the Problem of Being (way) Too Far Ahead of the Market

The year was 1983. I had a beautiful laboratory at the Bioengineering Center of Purdue, and six employees/collaborators working on a wearable dialysis ma- chine with ultimate simplicity. The Sorbent Suspension Reciprocating Dialyzer (SSRD) had round, flat sheet membranes with a single, central blood entry and return point.[12] It used a thick sorbent suspension as dialysate, to remove uremic toxins directly across the dialyzer membranes from the blood. Eli Lilly, sponsor of the project, had failure of one of their premier drugs in the market (Oraflex) and as a result pulled funding from all outside laboratories, including ours. On suggestion from one of my collaborators, I met Bob Truitt. He had an MBA from Harvard and Master of Engineering degree from Purdue University, and had decided that he would like to help scientists and engineers at Purdue to form spin-off companies.

Bob was fascinated by our research directions and wondered if there was a product around which we could form a company. At the Hemodialysis Lab we had already determined that a standard flat plate dialyzer with nonwoven screen supports could operate to pump blood and mix a dialysate sorbent suspension. Therefore, we could use a commercially available dialyzer with a sorbent sus- pension, to create a dialysis machine with many advantages of the SSRD. When used with a charcoal suspension it could treat drug overdose and liver failure, and with a sorbent column like the Redy™ Sorb™ it could treat kidney failure. Either way we would keep some of the simplicity of design of the SSRD, especially the pumping of blood by the dialyzer membranes at controlled pressures through a single access.

The Redy™ machine was already being used in home dialysis in many locations (especially Australia) because it required only 6 liters of potable tap water to perform a dialysis procedure. The clinical results and benefits of home dialysis with the Redy™ system were equivalent to that with a standard proportioning-system dialysis machine[13,14]. However, the Redy™ machine was crude by the dialysis standards of the 1980s. Most notably, it did not even have controlled ultrafiltration (UF) rate. We knew we could create a better machine.

So, in 1983 Bob Truitt and his wife Patti met with me and my wife Marianne and we all decided to create Ash Medical Systems. We established a Board mostly of Bob's contacts within the medical device, investment, and manufacturing industries. Bob raised an initial investment in the company which in retrospect seems modest, about $250,000. And, we were off...

Development of the BioLogic-HD™ (as we called it) progressed very well. We learned how to make the cellulosic plate dialyzers operate as a blood pump and how to control the UF rate. The Sorb company (who supported the Redy™ machine) supplied our columns and gave us technical information about them.

Our research group was largely made of recent graduates of Purdue schools of Engineering and Technology, such as Terry Echard and Kevin Sweeney. plus some as- sorted chemists and a pharmacologist. They were a hard-working and highly skilled group. I defined a dialysis machine technology with everything that I felt possible, to make dialysis simple, safe and well-suited for the home. The BioLogic-HD™ included:

    a. The Sorb column for regeneration of dialysate
    b. Dialysate created with 3 liters of potable tap water
    c. A commercial pyramidal-support plate dialyzer (from Gambro®)
    d. Automated ammonium monitor for dialysate
    e. Highly simplified blood circuit (no drip chambers or roller pump segments, the dialyzer served as the blood pump, and the circuit was airless)
    f. Pressure-actuated blood flow
    g. Single-needle operation
    h. A pre-assembled cartridge containing all disposable components
    i. Measurement of total fluid balance of the patient (with a scale measuring the entire top part of the machine)
    j. Ultrafiltration control

k. Direct measurement of blood flow rate

l. Highly portable size

m. An external power source with a battery capable of operation for 30 minutes

n. A hand-held module for displaying machine information and for control of the machine function.

All of this, it may be hard to believe, was completed in 1985[15]. To measure the blood flow rate, we first created a flow meter based on optical scattering of the blood, developed on research done at another university. Unfortunately we could never get the device to determine more than whether blood was moving or not. So, we took a "fallback" position and used the scale to detect changes in weight of the top part of the machine on inflow vs. outflow.

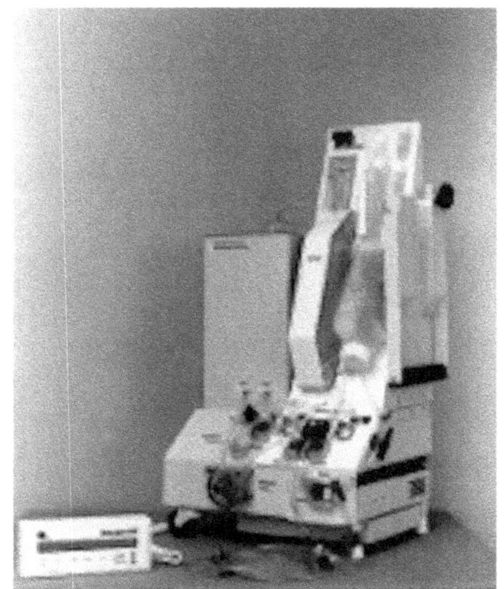

Figure 4. The BioLogic-HD™, a sorbent based, single access dialysis system, flat plate dialyzer membranes as the blood pump, controlled UF rate and automated fluid administration (1987).

Overall, our cost estimate for our development was way short of what it took. Bob raised some more money from investors and we applied to the NIH SBIR program to fund the final development of the machine. The review committee actually came to our small company for an on-site review, and approved the $500,000 grant we requested.

We met with the FDA and pointed out that the major components of this machine were already marketed, such as the plate dialyzer and the sorbent column and blood tubing. The new components like the ammonium detector just replaced a procedure done manually by Redy™ patients. We had well-written documentation of the ma- chine, extensive in vitro testing and a 510(k) application with an appropriate pred- icate (the Redy™ System). An important part of our data justified the omission of all filters and drip chambers in the blood circuit. Steve Badylak (then a PhD candi- date) evaluated particulate release in hemodialysis circuits using ultrasound signals and showed that there are more particles in blood leaving a drip chamber and filter than entering it.[16]

In 1986 the FDA approved the BioLogic-HD™ for marketing in the treatment of kidney failure. We began production of 20 of our home dialysis machines (Figure 4).

We completed a short clinical trial in our dialysis unit, showing that the machine func- tioned as expected, including UF control and measurement of blood flow rate by ma- chine weight changes.[17] Then we placed the first dialysis machine in a patient's home. It worked great, although there were bothersome alarms due to inaccuracies of our blood flow measurement. The blood flow measurement had worked beautifully in our clinic with a solid floor but in the patient's home the machine sat on a rug, decreasing scale accuracy. Our plan was to implement ultrasonic flow probes on the blood lines.

In the acute market we tested the machine on a few patients, and the treatments went fairly well in hospitals with the help of Kathryn Peters RN. Physicians and nurses weren't keen about a system that dialyzed slower than standard dialysis ma- chines but did realize that a single needle access and a slower treatment would have benefit for many patients. A more bothersome problem was occasional clotting of the dialyzer. The pH of the dialysate bath was quite low at the start of dialysis due to high pCO2 levels, in spite of bicarbonate in the dialysate. This acidity contributed to clotting of the dialyzer, which could have been avoided by increasing the heparin load, but the tendency to clotting was a second negative for the machine.

Overall the machine functioned well and had numerous features new to dialysis. However, we were unable to interest the few companies making dialysis machines for the US market in a radically different type of machine just for home use. Over- heard at one ASN meeting was a comment by a company representative "don't worry about them, they'll never make it."

At the time of our FDA approval, there were approximately 4000 home dialysis patients in the US and the number was steadily growing. Most of these patients were supported by "home helpers," with modest hourly payment by HCFA.[19] In 1987 HCFA made an announcement that they had found some double-billings by one company employing home helpers and in response, HCFA cancelled the home helper program altogether. Additionally, they announced that they would soon eliminate "Method II" payments, in which companies could bill for providing the supplies and machines for home dialysis and charge HCFA directly. In the course of a few months, almost all the home dialysis patients transferred to in-center units, leaving only 400 at home. All of a sudden, our principal goal market was gone!

At this time our company was being supported by a trio of venture capital funds, one from Indianapolis, one from Chicago and one from Texas. At our Board meeting, they stated that they would no longer support the company. The fact that the machine needed a little more development was a small part of their decision. As their principals left our Board meeting, we asked what they thought we should do. They said "turn it into an artificial liver." We were heart-broken. The next day we released about two- thirds of our twenty employees, many of whom were close friends. The Bio-Logic- HD™ machine was never marketed.

LESSONS LEARNED
A. It is hard to find an industrial partner for a product that is radical and revolutionary, even if it has highly beneficial new features.
B. Venture capital funds are vital to a small company, but venture capitalists are driven more by what they see as the market than by the benefits of the new technology.
C. When a single payor exists in a market, especially a governmental agency, policies can suddenly change and drastically alter the market.
D. Marketing a device perfectly suited for home dialysis but not really suited for in-center dialysis or acute dialysis is a hard sell to companies with established products, and to physicians familiar and comfortable with incenter dialysis.
E. Always choose the best technology for each task in a device, rather than the least expensive (as we did in choice of flow monitoring technology).
F. Realize that the first few patients treated during a Beta site evaluation of a new device must have a completely positive outcome for the physicians involved to become advocates.
G. Even after a device is patented, produced, shown to be effective and safe, and FDA approval is in hand, successful marketing of the device is not assured.

Chapter 4

The BioLogic-DT™ and the Saga of Liver Dialysis™

Everyone knows that necessity is the mother of invention. But few people ask "who is the father?" I can tell you, frustration is the father. Throughout my training and practice I would sometimes be asked to dialyze a patient with hepato-renal failure, but I quickly learned that these patients became worse on standard hemodialysis. standard hemodialysis.[20] Their coma did improve somewhat with hemoperfusion, in which blood is passed through a column of uncoated or coated charcoal granules, but the biocompatibility of the charcoal columns was so poor that adverse reactions and platelet removal limited most patients to a few days of treatment. I decided that hemodialysis failed in these patients because its removal of toxins was unselective whereas charcoal was selective. Charcoal binds aromatic amino acids better than branched-chain amino acids, and nonpolar organics better than polar organics. Hepatic toxins apparently could dissociate enough from the blood proteins to pass across the porous membrane and bind to the adjacent carbon during hemoperfusion. However, the rate of removal decreased after the first half-hour or so, as the carbon just beneath the membranes began to saturate with the toxins being bound.

The solution to both of these problems was to use a thick suspension of very small carbon particles, and mix them effectively at the membrane surface opposite the blood. This could provide a huge surface area for toxin removal, with continuous replenishment at the membrane surface, similar to our SSRD wearable dialyzer.[21] In the Bio- Logic-HD™ we utilized a plate dialyzer in which the blood compartment was expanded and then compressed by changes in dialysate pressure, to pump the blood.[22] A dialysate pump circulated dialysate from a small reservoir, through the dialyzer and then through the Sorb column to remove toxins of kidney failure. In order to treat liver failure patients, we designed the BioLogic-DT™. In it a 2-liter volume of a thick (7%) sorbent suspension containing powdered carbon was circulated through the plate dialyzer (Figure 5). Vacuum and pressure were applied to the sorbent suspension in a chamber. This pulled the sorbent suspension out of a bag, propelled it through the dialyzer and pushed it back to the bag. The back-and-forth motion of the plate membranes served to perfectly mix the sorbent suspension at the membrane surfaces, maintaining continued clearance of creatinine, drugs and hepatic toxins for up to 12 hours of use.

My business partner and good friend at Ash Medical was Bob Truitt. Our Bio-Logic-HD™ machine was not to be marketed, since our VC investors "walked" from the company after HCFA cut support for home dialysis helpers. Bob decided to transfer our sorbent and dialysis technology to a new company, which he cleverly called "HemoCleanse". He offered HemoCleanse stock to the shareholders of Ash Medical and they came through with sizeable investments, believing in Bob (and me too, I guess). Bob also offered HemoCleanse stock for purchase to the VC investors, but they turned down the offer, as Bob knew they would. So, we were totally free from VC involvement, and the brand-new company HemoCleanse was free to pursue the liver machine without their interference.

So, off we went again. We put the remaining employees to work in converting the "HD" machine to the "DT" machine. There were numerous R&D projects we needed to define each part of the machine: disposables, operating cycles, UF measurement, warming method, blood leak system, and user interface. All of these required extensive testing.

The development went well, and soon we began testing the machine on animals, to study biocompatibility and efficacy in models of liver failure. The first tests were performed at the U. of Pittsburgh in the lab of Dr. Leonard Makowka, with Dr. William Clark manning the machine. Animal tests in animals with surgically-induced liver failure were done

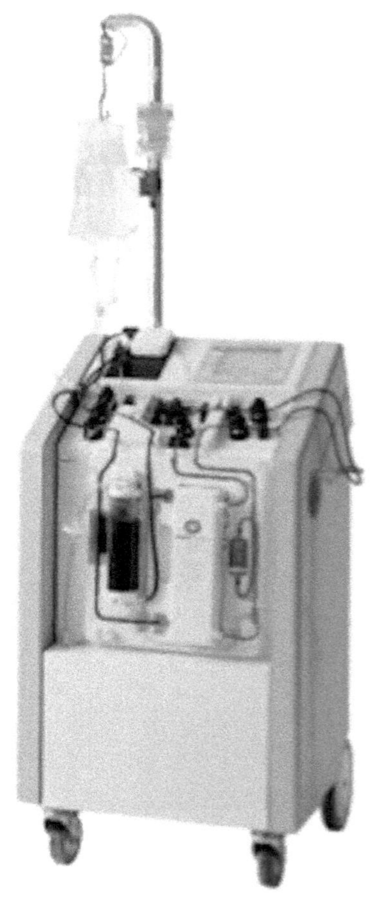

Figure 5. The BioLogic-DT™ (Liver Dialysis™) machine for treatment of liver failure and drug overdose. A thick sorbent suspension was propelled through the plate dialyzer, which served also as the blood pump. A 2 liter bag of sorbent suspension is behind the door at the left.

at Vanderbilt in the lab of Dr. Achilles Demetriou and Dr. Jacek Rozga, in a comparison to their bioartificial liver device. From our analysis of data, the BioLogic-DT™ effectively corrected abnormal physiology and chemistry of the animals.[23]

With considerable in vitro and animal testing data in hand, we met with the device division of FDA. We outlined clinical trials which would demonstrate safety and efficacy in patients with hepatic failure and coma. We proposed a prospectively randomized trial of treatment in patients with hepatic coma due to acute-on-chronic OR acute liver failure (stratified). Patients would be assigned to receive treatment with the DT device or standard of care treatment. Endpoints were to be improvement of coma, improvement in physiologic state, and outcome (recovery of liver function, support of the patient until transplantation, or death).

Staff were trained in operation of the machine and patients were recruited at several top liver transplant centers in the US. Through persistence we finally accumulated the proscribed 20 patients in the study, and Carol Gingrich RN served as clinical coordinator and trainer. When we analyzed the results, they showed definite improvement in coma level in the treated patients, especially those with acute- on-chronic liver failure, compared to the control group. The treatment improved the ratio of branched-chain to aromatic amino-acids.[24] Physiologic status improved (blood pressure and respiratory function). Renal status improved in those with significant hepato-renal failure, something that almost never happened with hemodialysis. Outcomes of the treated patients were significantly better but the main difference was that a higher percentage of patients who were treated by the machine received a liver transplant.[25] In parallel clinical trials in other centers, we showed that system functioned very well in removal of drugs from patients with significant overdose, especially valuable for patients with serious acetaminophen overdose and early signs of liver failure, or severe cases of tricyclic overdose.[26,27]

During a poster presentation of the clinical results of our trial at a scientific meeting, a key member of the CDRH section that had approved our clinical trial asked, "so when are you coming back to the FDA?" With the results of the clinical trial, we met with FDA and received approval to market the BioLogic-DT™ as a liver support system, with the following indications: Hepatic encephalopathy (due to fulminant hepatic failure or acute-on-chronic liver failure) and Drug Overdose and Poisonings (with drugs which are dialyzable and bound by charcoal).

Around this time, I had a visit from two bright young residents in Medicine from Rostock, Germany, Jan Stange and Steffen Mitzner. Having studied with Prof. Horst Klinkmann they were very interested in treatment of hepatic failure. During two days, I showed them exactly how our machine worked, and explained why sorbent-based dialysis had great potential in treatment of liver failure.[28] Their concepts and ideas eventually became the MARS™ system. Instead of using powdered charcoal as a sorbent on the dialysate side, they used albumin in dialysate to bind toxins, and then per- fused the albumin solution through sorbent columns to remove the toxins of liver failure. They had the advantage of using a high permeability hollow-fiber dialyzer membrane, something that we found would not work in the BioLogic-DT be- cause of stagnation of the sorbents contacting the membranes. In concept however, the two systems were similar, and the sorbents served merely to increase diffusion gradients for toxins across the dialyzer membrane, as shown in a publication by Jack Patzer PHD[29]. The MARS™ system was later shown to have good clinical benefit, especially in acute-on-chronic liver failure.[30,31,32]

To carry the BioLogic-DT™ to the market was a significant challenge. We needed a dedicated machine with pneumatics and specialized sensors for control of sorbent and blood flow (including an improved blood flow measurement system). Contract device manufacturers would have to produce the machine and dis- posable kits. A consistent supply of plate dialyzers with screen plates was needed, and only one company, Cobe was making them. Marketing, sales and support for new kind of extracorporeal therapy for hepatic failure would be a large task.

Bob and I decided that the best approach was to form a "spin-off" from Hemo-Cleanse to pursue the marketing and sales of the new liver failure treatment. Mr. Dave Mazepink of San Diego had consulted with HemoCleanse in marketing of some other products, and he was convinced that he could raise capital in Southern California to support a company marketing "Liver Dialysis." HemoCleanse agreed to license the DT machine to the company formed by Dave and some investors. They called the company HemoTherapies (somewhat reminiscent of HemoCleanse). In the agreement, HemoCleanse engineers and scientists would be in charge of finalizing the production version of the machine, creating the user inter- face and manuals, and supervising the contract medical device manufacturers for production of the machine and disposables, validation and verification. HemoTherapies would be responsible for all marketing and sales activities.

The marketing plan which HemoTherapies devised was logical and focused. There were already five liver transplant centers in the US which had utilized the DT system with some success in treating patients with liver failure. The marketing plan would first focus on these five centers, promote treatments for many patients with hepatic failure, and assure that doctors and nurses were satisfied with the out- comes. However, as venture capital groups became bigger investors in HemoTherapies, the focus changed to a much more aggressive plan to introduce the machine to many hospitals across the US, a "shotgun" approach. Machines and disposables were provided on a per-treatment charge (which was quite high). Soon over fifty hospitals in the US had used the machine, and many of the first patients treated were those with little hope of recovery of liver function or receiving a liver trans- plant. Education of centers became spotty at best. For example, the DT treatments worked best with a single lumen ten French multi-hole femoral catheter. HemoTherapies did not offer this catheter for sale, and did not emphasize its importance.

Making matters worse, the HemoTherapies company decided to ignore the overseas market. HemoCleanse had assisted physicians overseas in performing clinical trials of the DT system in patients with liver failure in Japan, China, Taiwan and Europe. HemoTherapies provided no further support for these trials with sup- plies or education. One study performed in Austria showed a moderate benefit in coma status for patients with acute-on-chronic liver failure, but three patients developed diffuse intravascular coagulation during the treatments.[33] This may have been due to the use of a double-lumen catheter instead of our low resistance single-lumen catheter, resulting in high shear stress on the blood.

Slowly, the enthusiasm of several centers turned to skepticism regarding the benefits of Liver Dialysis. When HemoTherapies finally realized that marketing this device was not going to be easy they decided to declare bankruptcy in 2000. Amazingly, they immediately sued HemoCleanse, demanding that our company relinquish rights to the DT technology to them so that it could be re-licensed. The lawsuit took a year or more to resolve, and the final verdict was in favor of HemoCleanse. HemoTherapies paid a large sum for damages to HemoCleanse, and HemoCleanse kept the technology. However, the reputation of "Liver Dialysis" had been tarnished. The technology was by this time "old fashioned", including the plate dialyzer that was central to its operation. Bob and I saw no hope for us to re- market the DT system, so the project ended. Two related projects also ended. One was the (DTPF) add-on module of Liver, in which a sorbent suspension surrounded plasma filter membranes and removed cytokines in treatment of sepsis and SIRS.[34] The other was an adaptation of the BioLogic-DT™ to use in whole body hyperthermia to remove toxins of kidney and liver failure and control serum calcium and phosphate levels.[35,36,37]

LESSONS LEARNED

A. When growing up, I always wanted to be first in anything I did. But having a first-in-class device like Liver Dialysis makes you run straight into a wall of skepticism, especially from "experts" in current therapies. It's much easier to be second-in-class with a better device.

B. Even if your first-in-human device doesn't make remain in the market, your device and its clinical success have been important, and you can feel justified when similar devices have clinical success (such as the MARS device, in our case).

C. Clinical trials of extracorporeal life support devices are complex and stressful, especially if patients are randomized to treated and control groups.

D. Most fatal illnesses involve highly complex interplay of various organ systems, and each patient is different, so clinical trials must be large and well stratified to be convincing.

E. FDA approval to market is no guarantee of market success of a new product, or company success.

Chapter 5

Allient™ Hemodialysis Machine;
Sorbent-Based, Single-Needle Sorbent Dialysis Reborn

During the 1990s, there was a stabilization of hemodialysis technology. Some would say it was more of a crystallization. The technologic improvements of the 1970s and 1980s had been implemented within the in-center units: controlled filtration, hollow fiber membranes, bicarbonate dialysate, easily adjustable concentrations of sodium and bicarbonate in the dialysate, high flux membranes, and blood volume measurements (with Crit-Line® for example). Using urea kinetics as a guide, treatment durations were shortened so that they fit the operations of the in- center dialysis units, less than four hours for most patients in the US. However, the mortality of dialysis patients in the US, especially from cardiovascular diseases was quite high. By comparison, patients in Japan and in some units in Europe had much lower mortality, which was apparent by the late 1990s. Led by Robert Lockridge and John Moran in the US and Bernard Charra in France, nephrologists began to realize that outcome results are much better if hemodialysis were performed on a more frequent schedule, or for a longer period of time.[38] The improvement in patient health with these schedules suggested that hemodialysis was the right tool to treat kidney failure all along, but our prescription of the treatments was all wrong.

I was telling Bob Truitt about the resurgence of interest in home dialysis, due to the potential for much better outcomes. This was in the year 2000. He said, "it's a shame we don't still have the BioLogic-HD™.[39] Maybe we should resurrect it. Do you think it could be designed with all new components?" I said "Sure we could." Then I remembered that capacity of sorbent columns for ammonium was increased by high dialysate urea levels and a slow dialysate flow rate. This was a perfect match for overnight dialysis. So, I said something like "And we should!" And thus started a new episode in our lives, the creation of Renal Solutions, Inc. and the Allient™ dialysis machine.[40]

I went back to my office and thought what "new components" meant. First of all, we had to utilize dialyzers with hollow fiber membranes rather than a plate dialyzer (since plate dialyzers had been replaced by hollow fibers). We also needed highly accurate measurement of blood flow rates, and a more graphic and instructive user interface. But there were many features of the BioLogic-HD™ that we really wanted to save:

- Sorbent regeneration of dialysate to allow dialysis with small volumes of tap water
- Automated ammonium monitoring to detect column saturation.
- Pressure-actuated blood flow, to eliminate pressure alarms, prevent over pressurization of the blood, eliminate the need for pressure gauges, and create a smooth blood flow profile
- Single-needle operation, changeable to more efficient dual-needle operation when desired
- Airless blood side circuit
- Automatic priming, rinsing and fluid administration
- Automatic UF control
- Completely disposable and pre-assembled blood and dialysate side tubing and the dialyzer.

The use of hollow fiber membranes meant that the dialyzer membrane compliance would be near zero, so using the membranes of the dialyzer to pump blood was out. Another type of pressure-controlled blood pumping was needed. Thinking of the artificial hearts I had seen in Utah and at each meeting of ASAIO, I decided that having two pumping chambers with flexible diaphragms would be the ideal blood pump. If both ventricles worked in unison, then the pumping would be perfect for single-access dialysis. Both ventricles would fill blood and then expel the blood in unison through the dia- lyzer and back to the patient. For dual- needle

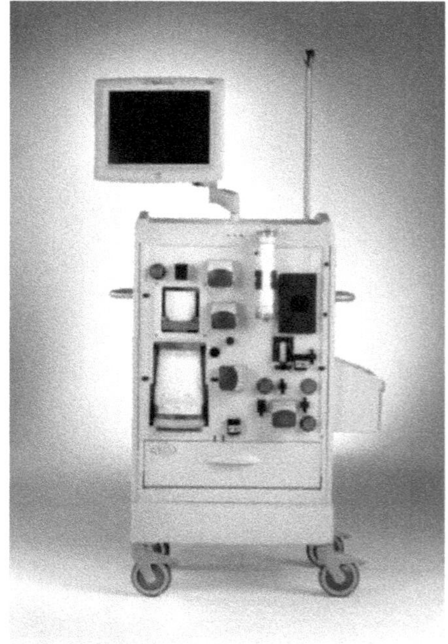

Figure 6. Allient™ hemodialysis machine, with sorbent regeneration of dialysate and pressure- controlled veentricles for single- and dual-access blood pumping.

access, when one ventricle was filling with blood, the other would be emptying, creating a nearly continuous flow of blood through the dialyzer. Active valves on inflow and outflow lines side would make the blood flow unidirectional, and allow the flow direction to reverse during dialyzer priming.

I laid out the projects that were needed: improved ammonium monitor, accurate blood flow meters (ultrasonic), and a computer program to direct choice of the proper Sorb® column, to match chemical function of the column with patient parameters and to define the starting dialysate composition. The improved user interface should provide easy-to-follow instructions for training staff and patients in machine set-up and operation, and relevant data during treatments. We would need improved sorbent columns, able to handle removal of urea for a complete overnight therapy, for almost any patient. And finally, we needed a new machine, filled with electronics, sensors, processors, and pneumatics (Figure 6).

Bob and I decided to create another spin-off company. The first decision was to find an effective CEO. Pete DeComo had been CFO for HemoTherapies, and his financial analyses and straight-forward assessment of progress helped the company raise millions of dollars. Pete and his family lived in Pittsburgh, PA and he found commitments both from the State and some highly supportive VC groups. So, Pittsburgh it was!

Pete named the new company Renal Solutions, Inc (RSI), and hired an experienced director of R&D (John Maholtz) and a nurse with extensive dialysis experience (Debbie Brouwer). He soon realized that the future of RSI and Sorb Technology were closely linked. Sorb Technology was the company that had originated the Sorb™ column in the 1970s for the Redy™ machine, and they continued to produce it in their facility in Oklahoma City. The company had previously been owned by Marquardt (an aerospace firm), CCI Life Systems, Organon Teknika and Gambro, before becoming a stand-alone company in 1999.[41] However, they had not had a new machine since the Redy 2000 was introduced in the 1980s, and that machine lacked controlled filtration (a very important and standard feature of almost all dial- ysis machines). RSI had a revolutionary dialysis machine, but no sorbent columns. Pete orchestrated the merger of RSI with Sorb, gaining the valuable expertise of staff there such as Preston Thompson, PhD.

Pete's team called the new machine, the Allient™. The development of the Allient™ began and proceeded well. RSI was in charge of hardware development, machine design and software to operate the machine, including the algorithms for measuring the amount of ultrafiltration and algorithms to adjust the UF rate. With scales and software to include the weight of the column, dialysate bag and Ca/Mg infusate, the system could measure the net fluid removal and UF rate accurately. RSI was responsible for designing the ultrasonic flow meters for inflow and outflow blood lines. These would assure that the blood flow rate through the ventricle pumps was consistent, and detect sudden changes as occur with occlusion of flow through the needle or catheter. The visual user interface for instruction and inputs and displays were developed with the direction of Debbie Brouwer and the engineers.

Sorb was assigned to create sorbent columns suited for overnight treatments and they would be larger than the old Sorb columns.. When Sorb joined RSI, the company was already developing columns with improved capacity and much more stable dialysate concentrations of sodium and hydro-gen. For the Allient™ four new column sizes and types were developed, each of which pro-duced less acidosis of the dialysate at the be-ginning of treatment, and a lower amount of sodium return to the patient.[42] The starting dialysate volume was six liters, similar to the Redy™ not three liters as in the BioLogic-HD™. Preston Thompson and Steve Merchant, a biochemist, led the effort to improve the col-umn function and suitability for all patients.

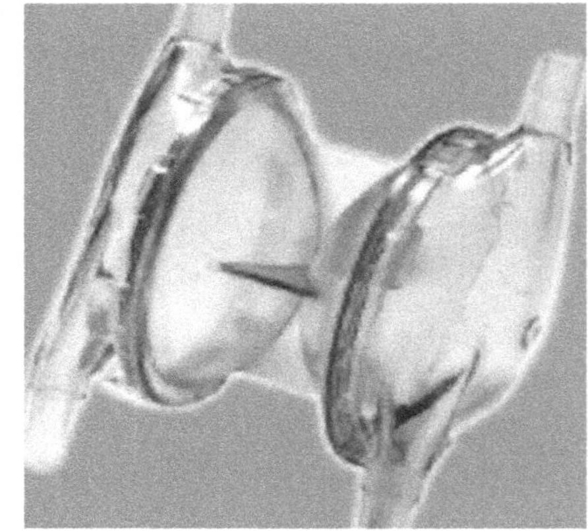

Figure 7. Dual ventricle pressure-actuated blood pump of the Allient™ hemodialysis machine.

HemoCleanse engineers built the automated ammonium detector, comparing three possible technologies. A "Therapy Calculator" program was developed, predicting the capacity of the column for ammonium and proper dialysate flows to avoid ammonium break- through, based on simple inputs such as patient weight, a recent BUN level, and desired treatment length. The program suggested the proper column to use, the desired dialysate flow rate, and the proper starting dialysate concentrations of chemicals.[43] The reliability of the predictions were confirmed by ex- tensive in vitro testing, and the results were pleasingly reproducible. However, as expected when regenerating a small dialysate volume by sorbents, the net removal or transfer of any chemical could be controlled, but the dialysate concentrations could not remain constant (as with proportioning dialysis machines). We determined safe ranges for dialysate concentrations in sorbent-based dialysis from the wide clinical experience with the Redy™ machine. The logic of this approach was later af- firmed in an AAMI Technical Information Report.[44]

The development of the blood pump and clamping components was assigned to a bioengineer named Dan Wellington in Rochester, New York. He designed a rugged and quite effective two-chamber pumping system. Each ventricle had its own membrane and inlet and outlet ports as shown in Figure 7. The pump worked well in the laboratory, and also in later clinical trials, but at the end of some patient treatments there were small clots in the pumping chambers after dialysis. The design was improved by Fangjun Shu and James Antaki in the Bioengineering Department of Carnegie Mellon University. Making the inlet port tangential to the chamber created circular motion, and using a pre-molded domed diaphragm emptied the chamber more evenly.[45]

Soon there was a workable machine prototype with most of the necessary features. By 2005, the machine was completed and validated. Renal Solutions approached FDA with an application for 510(k) approval, based on two predicates, Redy™ 2000 and BioLogic-HD™. The response of FDA was cordial and helpful, and they saw no technical problems with the machine. In 2006 the machine was approved by the FDA to market for treatment of kidney failure, "in the presence of a healthcare practitioner." The latter restriction was to indicate that the Allient™ was not to be used yet in home hemodialysis without a skilled technician or nurse being present. The FDA had already decided that there were extra safety requirements for machines to be used in home hemodialysis. Safety of devices for home dialysis use should be demonstrated in a clinical trial of about twenty patients. RSI completed production of 20 Allient machines and began clinical trials of dialysis outpatients and beta site evaluations in treatment of hospitalized patients. Published results of the clinical trials showed successful function of the machine and sorbent columns.[46]

In 2007 FMC announced that they were purchasing RSI (including the Sorb company). The purchase price in total (with payment for milestones) was about $200M. This payment resulted in a significant dividend to the 300 or so shareholders of HemoCleanse. But more important to me was that FMC was serious about creating a machine that was designed to fit the needs of home hemodialysis patients. I felt bolstered by their apparent understanding of the great benefits to home dialysis patients that would derive from sorbent regeneration of dialysate, and single access.

Soon there were some announcements by FMC that troubled me. They decided that the FDA-approved Allient™ needed a complete re-design, to make it smaller and more convenient to use. Amazingly, the RSI engineers who had worked with us on the machine wouldn't be the ones to re-design the machine. Instead, FMC chose to work with a small company in California who had de- signed an attractive looking home machine, but that machine had conventional blood pumps and pressure gauges and was not sorbent-based. In my mind I saw many of the unique features of our beloved Allient™ machine disappearing. Even worse, I had no communication whatsoever with the new engineers assigned to this re-design. FMC directed RSI to place the twenty completed Allient machines in a dumpster and have them hauled away. Many of the staff were terminated, others started new projects.

The "Portable Artificial Kidney" project of FMC was placed under management of one engineer in FMC. Each time I would meet him, for example at an ASN meeting, I would ask how the project was coming. He always said "It's coming along well." I doubted that. I would point out that ultrafiltration measurement and control in a sorbent-based dialysis machine is not an easy process. A major goal of FMC chairman Ben Lipps was to make a sorbent-based dialysis machine that would fit the functional features and current standards for dialysis machines. They wanted capability for dialysate flow rates of 500 ml/min or more, and absolutely stable and selectable sodium and bicarbonate levels. Their market feedback said that nephrologists did not want to use a machine that didn't function just like current proportioning machines. One project at FMC was to create an add-on module for the 2008 machine which would include the sorbent column for regeneration of the dialysate effluent. The goal of FMC seemed to be how to expand capabilities of the 2008 ma- chine, rather than how to make home dialysis therapy more practical.

After some years, it was apparent that the "re-design" phase of the Allient™ machine into the PAK was going nowhere. Slowly, the project fizzled out, and after about ten years, the whole project was cancelled. The net result was that FMC "buried" the Allient™ and with it a machine specifically designed for use   in the home. There may be plans and directions of FMC for some use of sorbent dialysis for a home environment, but no one at FMC seems willing to talk about this. In the Introduction, the failure of the Allient™ project is ascribed to the phase of redesign.[47]

A. Standards of an industry develop when technologies are mature and stable. When radically new technology is implemented to provide new advan- tages, the new device won't look or work like every other device on the market, and won't perfectly meet the standards.

B. Experts in medical therapies know all about current therapies. They know almost nothing of the problems and benefits of new technologies. This is true of university professors, leaders of medical device companies, and many practicing physicians.

C. There are always "trade-offs" with any device, and advantages and disad- vantages of every technology.

D. Spin-off companies and licensees tend to distance themselves from the originators of the technology, to emphasize their own contributions even more.

E. Sorbent dialysis allowed treatment of patients in many "nontraditional" places such as homes, ICUs and even mobile hospitals. Creating the proper dialysis prescription required special training and attention by physicians. Although the Redy™ system was used widely around the world, FMC found that physicians would not use a sorbent-based dialysis machine if it didn't perform exactly like the machines they use now. What changed? We did.

Chapter 6

Zirconium cyclosilicate: an oral sorbent for potassium, four decades in the making

It was in 2000 when I received a call from Dr. John Sherman at Union Carbide. We had collaborated in the early 1980s on calcium-loaded synthetic zeolites for cation exchange in our wearable artificial kidney, a project that failed partly because zeolites were too soluble for use in dialysate regeneration or as oral sorbents.[48,49] John said "I've got it!" I said "You've got what?" He said "What you always wanted, a cation exchanger with preference only for monovalent cations like potassium and ammonium." John explained that after the failure of zeolites to meet the requirements of an oral sorbent, he began to work with a company "UOP" that was partly owned by Union Carbide. UOP had gained experience in molecular design of crystals with pores of precise size and charge. They had a crystal called ZS-9 (sodium zirconium cyclosilicate, or SZC), a cation exchanger with strong affinity for monovalent cations but virtually no affinity for divalent cations (Figure 8). As a crystal, it was essentially insoluble, and therefore there were no concerns about solubility of and safety of this sorbent.

In the 1980s I told John that if Union Carbide developed a selective sorbent for potassium I would test it as an oral sorbent in animals (for no charge). We had

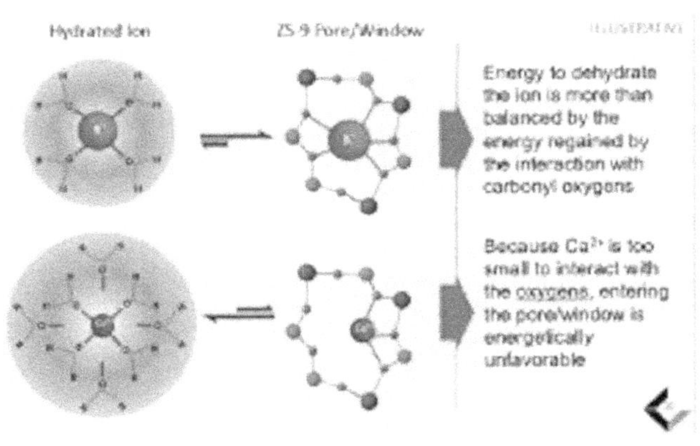

Figure 8. Zirconium Cyclo-Silicate, a crystalline cation exchanger with negatively charged pores which interact perfectly with potassium, but im- perfectly with calcium and magnesium.

performed studies of removal of uremic substances through the gut in the late 1970s using a "Roux-Y" intestinal bypass, so I knew how to measure the chemical binding of oral sorbents. [50] John sent a sample of SZC, and also invited me to participate in the first public presentation on SZC, an abstract to be presented at the ASAIO meeting in 2001.[51] Our own in vitro tests soon confirmed that sodium-loaded SZC had uniquely high selectivity for potassium and ammonium and almost no affinity for divalent cations.

I talked to Bob Truitt, my long-term business partner at HemoCleanse, about spending money on animal tests to study this brand-new potential oral therapy for hyper- kalemia. As usual we were short on cash, and working to form a spin-off Renal Solutions to reinvent the home dialysis machine.[52] To diminish expense, the animal trial would include just five normal adult rats in metabolic cages. A feed company pelletized rat food with SZC in it and we fed it to the rats, alternating with normal feed (5 days on and 5 days off). There were no signs of any toxicity in these animals. When we looked at the assay results of twenty-four-hour urine samples we were astounded. During the times of administration of SZC in the food, the urinary potassium didn't just decrease, it disappeared! Even during the five days of regular food ingestion, urinary potassium never re- turned to normal, but remained very low.[53] The function of SZC in removing potassium from the body was clearly much greater than that of the existing cation exchanger used as an oral sorbent, sodium polystyrene sulfonate (SPS, Kayexalate®). There was no removal of Ca++ or Mg++ from the body with SZC as there is with SPS. A surprising effect was that SZC removed significant amounts of urea from the body. Urea enters the gut from the blood and is quickly catalyzed to ammonium and bicarbonate by bacterial urease. SZC decreased urea excretion in the urine of our rats by about 30%, indicating that SZC in the gut removed urea from the body about as well as one normal kidney. There was however a significant transfer of sodium to the body of the rats and to the urine, in exchange for the bound ammonium and potassium.

Clearly we had a winner in this product. There was no oral sorbent that could predictably and rapidly decrease serum potassium levels in patients. But Union Carbide and UOP developed this product mostly for industrial use, not for medical use. The first thing that we needed to do was to obtain a license from UOP for SZC, for all medical uses. The next thing that we needed was to figure out how to load the SZC mostly with hydrogen, so that most of the exchange of ammonium would be for hydrogen rather than for sodium.

Our laboratory began working on the counter-ion problem, to determine how much we could load the SZC with hydrogen without reaching very low pH levels which degrade the sorbent. Bob worked on the licensing issue and also filed a provisional patent on SZC as an oral sorbent for potassium and ammonium.

UOP had a long history in catalyst chemistry, most of which I knew little about. UOP began as Universal Oil

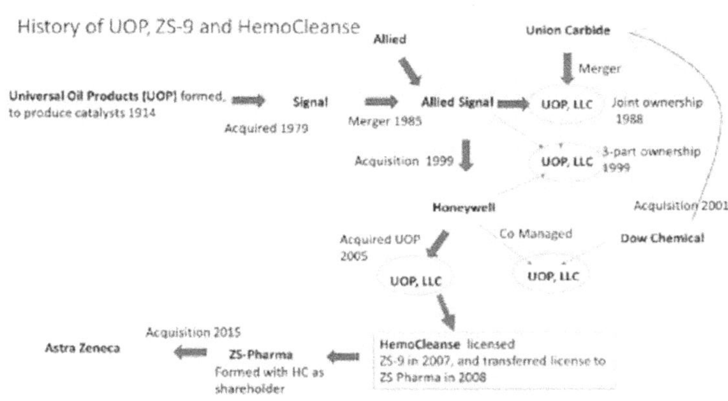

Figure 9. History of UOP, successive owners and the zirconium cyclo-silicate crystal technology

Products in 1914 to produce catalysts to create refined products like gasoline from crude oil (Figure 9). They were then purchased by Signal, which then merged with Allied to become Allied Signal. A flurry of other companies then had part ownership of UOP. In 2005 Honeywell spun off UOP as a limited liability company (LLC), and the Honeywell legal department called Bob about a license of SZC for medical uses. Deliberation on the license terms was finally completed in 2007. UOP had a number of patents protecting SZC and its methods of production, which went along with the license. In one of the early patents John Sherman had inserted a claim that SZC would be an excellent oral sorbent for binding potassium. His patent predated our provisional patent by a few weeks, so we no longer needed to pursue our patent.

Bob and I decided to create a spin-off, single-product company focused on SZC, called ZS Pharma. In exchange for the license of SZC as an oral sorbent, HemoCleanse received a sizeable amount of stock. Mr. Tim Opler helped to organize the company and find venture capital partners. We installed Al Guillem, PhD as manager of pro- duction and QA. Al had previously worked with our sister company Ash Access. He contacted Jeff Keyser, Pharm D who became CEO of the new company. ZS Pharma was located in the Dallas-Fort Worth area, home to Al and Jeff.

The principals in the company all contributed money to fund initial research ef- forts, and then worked without charge until the company found significant funding. Texas came through with a sizeable grant to help start the company. With significant funding from Venture Capital groups, and inclusion of an engineer from UOP, ZS Pharma began the effort to develop prototype production of SZC. Since SZC is a crystal, it had to be created at high temperatures and pressures, over many days, and scaling the process up was a significant challenge. HemoCleanse defined the steps needed to change the loading of SZC from pure sodium to mostly hydrogen and some sodium.

I estimated that for patients with hyperkalemia, the oral dose for SZC would be five or ten grams, once or more daily. Coming from the pharmacy industry, Al felt that the drug would be best given as pills. But since pills contain at most about one gram of a drug, some patients would be ingesting ten pills at one time! In the 1980s our laboratory developed a powdered calcium carbonate product for control of phosphate levels, and we found that patients with chronic kidney disease (CKD) were comfortable taking ten grams or more of the suspended powder orally. So, the first form of SZC was to be a dry powder suspended by the patient in a small amount of water.

ZS Pharma began planning numerous an- imal tests, and in pre- liminary meetings with FDA they defined the necessary pre- clinical data set. The animal tests were conducted very well, in several lo- cations. Efficacy was measured principally by changes in urinary ex- cretion as in our origi- nal study, confirmed by blood tests. After the first animal study, we

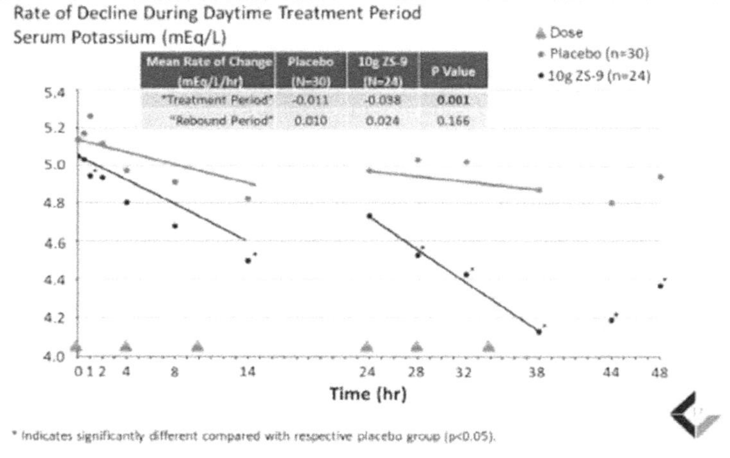

Mean Rate of Change (mEq/L/hr)	Placebo (N=30)	10g ZS-9 (N=24)	P Value
"Treatment Period"	-0.011	-0.038	0.001
"Rebound Period"	0.010	0.024	0.166

Figure 10. Rapid and significant decrease in serum potassium levels in CKD patients ingesting 10 grams of SZC powder three times daily (from ASN presentation 2013, and reference 54)

realized that we should increase the hydrogen loading of the SZC compound a little further, since the urine became quite alkaline with administration of the sorbents. One surprising finding of the animal trials was that if the sorbent mixture was given by gavage injection it had almost no binding of potassium or any uremic toxins in the gut. However, it worked remarkedly well if given as a mixture with food. The reason for this difference was not clear, but may have been due to rapid transit of the sorbent through small bowel, induced by gavage injection.

Finally, we were ready to move to clinical trials. I helped to design the Phase II study, in which we would determine not only safety but a measure of efficacy in a dose-escalation format. Patients would be those with CKD and moderate potassium elevation. A blinded, randomized trial was made possible by finding a placebo product which mimicked the consistency of the SZC powder. I insisted that both control and treated groups obtain 24-hour urines to measure efficacy of the sorbent, as well as blood tests. FDA agreed with the trial design.

As in the animal trials, SZC would be administered without any laxative-inducing medications. Animal trials indicated that SZC administration did not change the bowel function of the animals. The data from the Phase II clinical trial demonstrated that the SZC product was clearly safe and produced few, if any GI side effects. Potassium binding by SZC was very effective. The 10-gram doses caused approximately 1 meq/L drop in serum potassium in one to two days (Figure 10). More surprising was the rapidity of action. At higher doses (ten grams) the powder created a small but significant drop in serum potassium one hour after ingestion.[54] This rapid action could only happen if the binding of potassium by SZC occurred in the small bowel. Because there is passage of electrolytes through intercellular slits of the small intestinal mucosa, the mucosa is "leaky" and functions very much like a dialyzer. The specific binding of potassium to SZC would create low concentrations in the small intestinal lumen and promote diffusion of potassium into the gut. In the colon, potassium is actively transported into the lumen. The concentration of potassium is very high at 50 to150 meq/L but the amount of potassium present in the water portion of stool is fairly small.[55,56] SZC binds potassium in the small bowel and colon, but SPS binds it mostly in the colon.

The Phase II study also showed that SZC had a beneficial effect on serum bicarbonate levels, an increase of 2-3 meq/L versus the control group. There were no signs of sodium loading of the patients. Apparently we had put just the right amount of hydrogen ion on the SZC. SZC also absorbed a significant amount of ammonium in the gut. Patients on the higher doses of SZC (10 grams three times daily) had a decrease of blood urea levels of about 20% over two days. This was somewhat surprising since the body incorporates about 7 grams of nitrogen into urea daily. A twenty % decrease in BUN due to intestinal sorption of ammonium would mean SZC in the gut (30 grams) bound about 90 meq of ammonium daily (3 meq/gram), higher than the ap- parent binding of potassium (about 1 meq/gram). ZS Pharma quickly moved to Phase III studies of SZC in patients with hyperkalemia due to CKD and cardiac failure (in which drug treatments can exacerbate hyperkalemia). The Phase III trials were very large, well done, and demonstrated the same efficacy and safety as shown in the Phase

II trials. [57] Probably the pinnacle of my career was my 2013 presentation on Phase II and III trials during the "Late Breaking Clinical Trials" session at American Society of Nephrology (ASN).[58] Several Phase III studies confirmed the mild increase in serum bicarbonate levels with SZC, and a later path analysis performed in a meta- analysis showed that the probable cause for this increase in bicarbonate was ammonium absorption by SZC in the gut. [59] The Phase III studies also confirmed that SZC decreased serum urea levels in a dose-dependent manner, with the highest doses causing a decrease of 15 to 20%.[60,61] In end-stage renal disease (ESRD) patients oral SZC can effectively decrease high pre-dialysis potassium levels in patients on 3/week dial- ysis.[62] In 2015 ZS Pharma presented results of all the clinical trials to the FDA. The FDA agreed that no more clinical data was required to demonstrate safety or efficacy of SZC in treatment of hyperkalemia. They did require a notice in the instructions for use that some patients at higher doses of SZC developed edema. The only remaining requirement for FDA approval was validation and verification of the production process. In late 2015 I learned through the press that ZS Pharma had been sold to AstraZeneca for $2.7 Billion, in cash.

The validation and verification of production of SZC took much longer than expected, so world-wide marketing of SZC as Lokelma® began in 2019. Market experience with Lokelma® has been gratifying. Numerous publications have appeared, showing benefit of treatment for hyperkalemia CKD patients, ESRD patients on he- modialysis, heart failure patients, and patients on angiotensin converting enzymes (ACEs), angiotensin receptor blockers (ARBs) or spironolactone medications.[63] After the first clinical trials, John Daugirdas MD predicted that using SZC in chronic hemodialysis patients would decrease the need for very low potassium levels in dialysate, and increase safety of dialysis. That has come to pass.

At the time ZS Pharma was sold, HemoCleanse owned less than one percent of ZS Pharma stock. Waves of investment from venture capital companies and individuals had significantly diminished our ownership. However, the sale still created a size- able payment to HemoCleanse from AstraZeneca. Bob suggested that we should disband the company and distribute the cash from sale of the company to the share- holders directly (many of whom had first invested in Ash Medical in the 1980s). I had several projects in the laboratory which were not complete, so I offered to purchase the laboratory equipment, supplies, and intellectual property related to sorbents through purchase of a subsidiary, HemoCleanse Technologies LLC. I continued re- search on these projects with the help of two engineers. One of our major projects is to design a sorbent to bind five small uremic toxins in the gut, including potassium, sodium, hydrogen, phosphate, and ammonium (from urea).[64] Our animal studies in the 1970s indicated that all of these toxins are plentiful in the gut and could be removed effectively by sorbents.[65]

A. From a business standpoint, creating a single-product spin-off from an R&D "skunkworks" is a great way to bring new expertise, energy, and funding to a project. However, this route always results in dilution of ownership and loss of control by the parent company.

B. What is important in all research is perseverance. As Winston Churchill said "Never give up. Never, never, never, never." It was over forty years ago that our laboratory collaborated with Union Carbide to find and test a selective cation exchanger for potassium. It took almost twenty years for SZC to progress from early animal trials to the market.

C. When a new product is transferred from an R&D company to a single-product company, the role of the originator/inventor is diminished at the single-product company. Expect this. Write your own history.

D. Before beginning animal trials, make sure that a product is as perfect as can be. Be willing to redesign the product when any issues are found. Then start clinical trials.

Chapter 7

The "Ash Split-Cath";
The Best Inventions are Simple

I remember my first experience in actually performing hemodialysis treatments, while a first-year fellow in Nephrology at Indiana University Medical Center in 1974. The patient had acute renal failure, and a second-year fellow (Dr. Alan Handt) showed me how to place Shaldon catheters in femoral veins and arteries to obtain blood access for the procedure. Using the Seldinger technique and finding the femoral artery pulse, I placed an 18 gauge needle in the artery and threaded the guidewire through it. We then advanced the Shaldon catheter over the guidewire and secured it in place. We then placed another catheter in the nearby vein. The Shaldon catheter was a long, straight, single lumen catheter with side-holes all around the tip.[66] It was fairly stiff so that it could be advanced over a guidewire. The catheters worked fine throughout the dialysis procedure and I thought "Hey, I can do this!" However, my elation was short lived, when at the end of the treatment we removed both catheters, since they would cause too much damage to the vein and artery if left in place. So, we placed two such catheters for each dialysis treatment of the patient. Sometimes we placed both catheters in the femoral vein, though these didn't work quite as well for blood outflow. Obtaining blood access for each dialysis treatment was a tedious process for me, and a stressful and somewhat painful procedure for the patient. I wished there was a more practical and painless blood access that could be placed that would last a week or more.

It was in the late 1970s that the first double-lumen "acute" central venous catheter (CVC) for dialysis were introduced, designed to be placed into the superior vena cava over a guide wire. The first of these by Dr. Robert Uldall had concentric lumens and the inner one was placed and removed each treatment. Then Dr. Sakharam Mahurkar invented a cylindrical tunneled catheter with two semicircular,

D-shaped lumens (DD, back-to-back), which was optimally placed through the right internal jugular (IJ) vein. This design provided low blood flow resistance, allowing higher blood flow rate than concentric catheters of the same size, and the catheter could be left in place for one week. Quickly, several companies began producing acute dialysis catheters with DD lumens, and I gladly began using them.

In the late 1980s, Wayne Quinton devised a "chronic" tunneled CVC for use in patients who were beginning hemodialysis therapy.[69] The "PermCath" had a oval body with two round lumens, one for blood outflow and the other for blood return to the body. A subcutaneous Dacron® cuff promoted fibrous tissue ingrowth, to provide catheter stability and prevent migration of bacteria around the catheter (adapted from Dr. Tenckhoff's peritoneal dialysis catheter). The tips were blunt and the body was soft, so there was much less irritation to veins than with the stiff and pointed "acute" dialysis catheters. The tips were staggered or "stepped" in position, with the blood outflow port "upstream" and the return port "downstream." Placement of the catheter through the internal jugular (IJ) vein was made possible through the newly-invented "split-sheath", a thin plastic sheath placed into the vein over a dilator. When the dilator was removed, the catheter was advanced through the sheath, and the sheath was split into two halves to allow passage of the cuff along the tract of the catheter. How- ever, placement of this oval catheter using the sheath was cumbersome, even through the right IJ, and many of the catheters were placed surgically.

In the early 1980s, Dr. Mahurkar applied the DD design to create a cylindrical tunneled dialysis catheter. The cylindrical shape made use of the split-sheath much easier. Quickly, several companies brought out tunneled dialysis catheters with DD lumens and stepped tips. I began to have them placed in my patients by radiologists and surgeons through the IJ approach, and thought that blood access problems for patients starting dialysis would soon be solved.

However, I soon found that the flow rates from the tunneled CVC tended to de- crease over time, so that they often needed to be replaced after two to four months of use. In the 1990s I was impressed with the long-term function of the Canaud-Tesio catheters used in Europe. These were actually two separate single-lumen catheters, one for blood outflow and the other for blood return to the body. Each catheter had a sub- cutaneous cuff (Tesio) or grommet (Canaud) to fix its position.[70] With proper placement of the tips within the right atrium and some maintenance procedures, these catheters could be used in home dialysis patients for years, not just months.[71] The Canaud-Tesio catheters had side-holes around the entire perimeter of the tip, and the tips lay in different parts of the SVC and right atrium. Since the end of each catheter was cylindrical in shape, blood could enter each lumen from all directions. In the single-body DD catheters side-holes could only be on one side for each lumen, because the other side of each lumen was the wall separating the lumens. If the side-holes rested against a vein or atrial wall, they could suck the wall over the lumens, obstructing outflow from the catheter. Obstruction worsened when a fibrous sheath developed around the catheter, holding it against the venous wall. With the Canaud-Tesio catheters, if holes on one side of a catheter lay against a vein wall, the holes on the other side could draw blood from the center of the vein.

Also with two separate catheters it was easier to assure that tips of each catheter were well within the right atrium, which was diffi-cult with stepped-tip catheters. When tips of the catheter are in the right atrium, they are less prone to be covered with a fi- brous sheath. 72

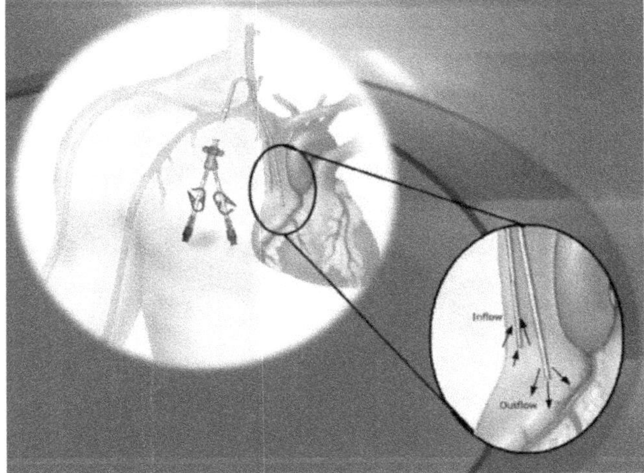

Figure 11. Ash Split Cath™ a tunneled and cuffed dialysis catheter with one body and two split tips.

I asked the surgeons and ra-diologists of our clinic about placing Tesio catheters, and they said that they didn't want to place these catheters because it would require placing each catheter individually. It was just "too much work." So I decided to start placing tunneled CVC myself. I had placed many acute CVC for dialysis, which became easier when ultrasound guidance became available. However, I needed supervision and training for placing a tunneled CVC. A surgeon with our clinic, Dr. David Barbara agreed to be my men-tor for the procedure. He did not use ultrasound for placement of the catheters, but I insisted that this was better for any type of CVC. After a couple of years, I had placed dozens of Tesio catheters under Dave's supervision and he said "You don't do it the same way I would, but your placements are safe and the catheters work."

At the start of my training in placing Tesio catheters I actually was glad that there were two catheters to place. It gave me twice the experience per placement. However, after placing many of these catheters, I began to agree with the surgeons and radiologists that placing two catheters rather than one was rather tedious. So I thought "why not have a catheter with a single body on the outside but with split tips at the end?" I went into the laboratory one day in the early 1990s. I took a scalpel and cut a single-body Mahurkar chronic catheter, about in the middle of the intravascular portion. I then cut the tips from two Tesio catheters and glued them onto the two lumens of the catheter. I had a visit the next day with a representative from Medcomp, the company which supplied our Mahurkar DD catheters. I showed her this new approach to dialysis access and she seemed to like the idea. I put the catheter model in an envelope and wrote a note on the outside to the President of the company Tony Madison, saying "Make This." He called back a week or so later, and with the help of my business partner Bob Truitt, a license agreement was made between HemoCleanse and Medcomp. Their chief engineer Tim Schweikert created the final design of the catheter, and Tony called me to see if it was Okay to call the catheter the "Ash Split Cath".[73] Very quickly this catheter became the most popular tunneled CVC for dialysis on the market world-wide, since it did provide somewhat better flow than the single-body catheters (Figure 11).

For several years, royalty payments to HemoCleanse from Medcomp were quite large. However, there were a number of competitive companies coming out with their own split-tip catheters. I had left writing the patent application to Medcomp, and they were quite impressed when their engineers had developed a way not only to make a split-tip catheter, but also to allow the user to decide how long the "split" should be. So, the patent that was created focused on a "splittable" catheter rather than a "split-tip" design. This allowed competitors to enter the market with catheters in which the tips were "split" but not "splittable." Royalty payments began to decrease, and on investigating the reasons, we realized that royalties were not being calculated by the formula we thought was outlined in the license agreement. The license agreement had specifically described that the royalty was to be calculated based on the "kit" price. The kit had been defined to include not only the catheter but all of the components needed to place it. Somehow, royalties paid to us were being calculated on the portion of the kit costs represented by the catheter. Our discussions with Medcomp became somewhat "polarized" to say the least. When Medcomp offered a fair buy-out for the remainder of the patent royalties, we decided that was the easiest course for all involved. A casualty of this dispute with Medcomp was the relationship we had developed between our two companies. Some years later I designed a split-tip catheter with two tips bending inward (CentrosFLO™) to avoid fibrous sheathing of the tips.[74] This catheter was licensed to another company, not Medcomp.

LESSONS LEARNED:

A. When deciding what major company to approach as a project partner for a new invention, choose a company with the closest product now in the market. They will have experience in design and production of this type of product and an effective sales force. This is especially important if the invention is an improvement of a product rather than a brand-new concept. Medcomp's excellent production and marketing of the Ash Split Cath was responsible for much of its success.

B. Successful marketing and widespread use of an improved product is easier than implementation of a whole new type of product. The split-tip catheter was really just an improvement of single-body dialysis CVC in the market.

C. Protect your intellectual property with a provisional patent before approaching major companies as a partner in the project. In the case of the Ash Split Cath, I was lucky.
Medcomp respected and recognized my rights as inventor, without any existing patent protection. However, if I had roughed out some kind of original description in a provisional patent, I would have been unlikely to substitute "splittable" for "split" in the regular patent application.

D. Regarding license agreements, make sure all words such as "product" and "kit" are carefully defined. Make sure that everyone agrees with the definitions, before signing the license agreement.

E. There are always several new technologies that intersect to enable a new invention. The ancestors of the Split Cath include acute and chronic double-lumen CVC such as the Quinton Perm-Cath, DD body catheters, Canaud-Tesio catheters, and the split-sheath.

F. Close personal experience with a product or procedure leads to the most important inventions. My frustration with the performance of dialysis CVCs in my own patients drove me to look for better solutions. But if I had not learned how to place Canaud-Tesio catheters myself, and then found that it was somewhat tedious, I would never have thought of combining single-body and twin catheters. In 2000 I joined Drs. Jack Work, Gerald Beathard and Charles O'Neill to form the American Society for Diagnostic and Interventional Nephrology (ASDIN) to encourage nephrologists to train in procedures and improve the care of patients with kidney disease.

G. If ultrasound machines had not come into use for real-time guidance during catheter placement, I would never have had the courage to place chronic or acute CVC for dialysis through the internal jugular approach. Improvements in new methods of imaging and new techniques also spur new inventions, directly and indirectly.

Chapter 8
Concentrated Sodium Citrate Catheter Lock; "The best laid schemes o' mice an' men..."[75]

My first frustration with "permanent" tunneled central venous catheters (CVC) for dialysis was that the flow was not permanent. Due to apposition of side holes with vein and atrial walls, and fibrous sheathing, many tunneled CVC for dialysis provided flow for a few months only. This led me to gain experience placing Canaud-Tesio catheters, and to develop the Ash Split Cath™ and eventually the Cen- trosFLO™ catheters.[76] But another major problem was even more catastrophic for patients, that of catheter infection. I hated it every time i had to remove a Split-Cath due to loss of flow or infection. In spite of the best efforts of nurses and patients, intraluminal contamination was causing catheter-related bloodstream infection (CRBSI) in many of our patients each year. Often the first sign of catheter infection was a fever which occurred during dialysis therapy, when the blood flow loosened bacteria from a biofilm within the catheter and they entered the bloodstream. These patients usually required hospitalization, antibiotic therapy and often removal of the CVC to prevent severe sepsis. Sometimes the infections were less obvious but much more serious, such as blood born bacteria that settled in a vertebra, a heart valve, or elsewhere. To prevent catheter infections, some physicians created mixtures of anti- coagulants with antibiotics to fill the catheter between uses (catheter locks). However, like almost all uses of prophylactic antibiotics, antibiotic catheter lock solutions would almost certainly result in emergence of antibiotic resistant bacteria in the patient and the population, so antibiotic catheter locks were not widely used.

In the process of developing the BioLogic-HD™, HemoCleanse wanted to make all the disposable components pre-attached and as simple to install as possible.[77] We wanted to provide the dialysate infusate of calcium-magnesium-potassium acetate as a premixed solution in a plastic bottle, rather than as dry powders as used in the Redy™ system. The bottle was to be one component of a cartridge which held all dis- posable components. We did not wish to have to sterilize the infusate solution, so it needed to be intrinsically antiseptic to avoid bacterial growth during storage of the cartridge. We performed bacteriologic studies to determine whether bacteria would grow in our highly concentrated salt solution and discovered that if the osmolality were about 1000 mOsm or more growth was inhibited for all common bacteria. This is why concentrated salt solutions are antibacterial.[78] So I wondered what kind of chemical might be an appropriate catheter lock solution and thought "Aha! Sodium Citrate!" Sodium citrate (Figure 12) is a known anticoagulant. It works because it binds calcium, which is a necessary cofactor of numerous blood clotting factors. Sodium citrate had already been used in 4% concentration as a catheter lock for patients who were known to be allergic to heparin or who had bleeding tendencies. Citric acid was known to be an effective antiseptic, but much of this effect was due to the low pH, which denatures proteins. We needed a catheter lock solution that had anti- bacterial properties, but did not degrade plasma proteins. So, I asked our biochemist Janusz Stezcko and pharmacologist Donald Blake at Ash Access to determine whether concentrated sodium citrate was itself antibacterial at pH near neutral.

What we found was encouraging. At concentrations of 7 to 10 %, sodium citrate had a modest antibacterial function. At concentrations of about 23 % the antibacterial function became quite significant, and even more so at 47%.[79] No bacteria we tested were resistant to the effects of concentrated citrate, and no resistance appeared after repeated exposure to citrate. Solutions of 4% sodium citrate are used as an anticoagulant during white blood cell separation and plasmapheresis procedures. Citrate is also often used during continuous veno-venous hemodialysis procedures performed in ICUs, as an anticoagulant, though this use is "off label." Vials with 30 ml of 47% sodium citrate are available for use in these procedures but they are diluted to 4% concentration before use.

One of the dialysis units associated with Ar- nett Clinic was in a lake resort town north of Lafayette. One summer the unit had a rash of CRBSI related to chronic

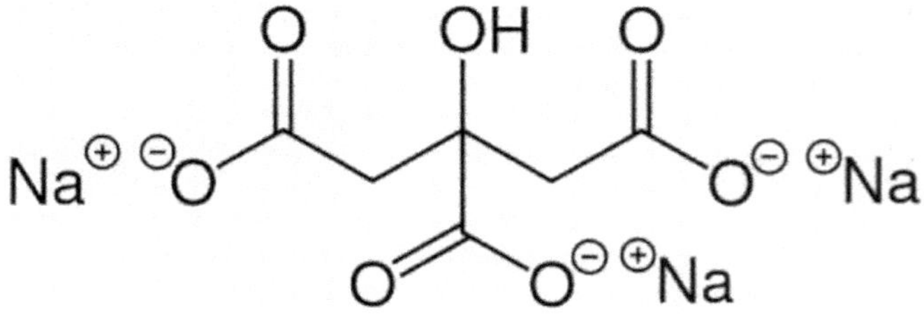

Figure 12. Structure of trisodium citrate. Calcium is bound more strongly than sodium.

CVC for dialysis, with an overall rate of up to 7 infections per 1000 patient-days. After discussions with nursing staff and observation of procedures failed to come up with a cause, I decided to offer use of concentrated sodium citrate as a catheter lock to patients who were concerned about the risk of infection. For three months we utilized 10% sodium citrate with 3 mg/ml gentamicin. The next four months we used 23% sodium citrate with 3 mg/ml gentamicin, and in the next three months 47% sodium citrate alone. Then we returned the patients to use of heparin for several months, and then used 23% sodium citrate as catheter lock. At the start of each portion of this study, I placed the new catheter lock solution myself, for each patient. Most patients reported feeling totally normal during administrations. About 10% of the patients did complain of a "metallic" taste in their mouth or tingling of the fingers shortly after the citrate catheter lock was placed.

It was during use of 47% sodium citrate that I realized that patients who were active would often return to the dialysis units for next treatments with blood having risen into the catheter extension set. This also happened with heparin catheter locks, just not as frequently. In laboratory tests I demonstrated that concentrated sodium citrate was falling out of catheters because the density of this solution was higher than that of blood. The effect was much less apparent with 23% citrate catheter lock.[5] Heparin with density lower than blood is displaced from the catheters, prob- ably whenever the patient is positioned so the tip is higher than the ports of the catheter. Some years later, Dr. Hans Polaschegg in Germany published a very nice paper demonstrating that in the laboratory, even very small differences in density between a locking solution and the surrounding blood would cause egress of the catheter lock solution from cylindrical lumens of simulated catheters.[80]

The antibacterial effect of the concentrated sodium citrate was encouraging. The incidence of positive blood cultures in the dialysis unit fell with use of the 10% solution with gentamicin, and decreased further with use of the 23% solution with gentamicin. With 47% solution (and without gentamicin) the infection rate for one month was zero. On returning the population to use of heparin for four months the positive blood cultures and CRBSI recurred. When using 23% sodium citrate lock solution again for five months (without gentamicin) the infections nearly disappeared.[5] Furthermore, the use of 23% sodium citrate lock greatly de- creased need for a clot-busting drug called TPA to restore patency of catheters, and 47% sodium citrate lock avoided the need for TPA altogether.

In our publication on this study we did not recommend use of 47% sodium citrate for locking dialysis catheters, due to the tendency to fall out of the catheters. In spite of the high efficacy shown in our clinical trials using 47%, we wrote that we "accepted 23% citrate as our standard locking solution" and we titled the publication "Concentrated Sodium Citrate (23%) for Catheter Lock".[5] In our original publication on concentrated sodium citrate as a catheter lock, we included an elaborate safety analysis, to determine what would be the expected toxicity from a citrate lock solution if, somehow, the sodium citrate lock was injected directly to the bloodstream. We predicted that 2 ml of 23 % sodium citrate would cause no symptoms at all. This was confirmed by rapid injection to a "normal" volunteer (guess who?). A review of animal studies in the literature showed that injection of ten catheter volumes (20 ml) of 23 % sodium citrate would be expected to cause only transient hypotension and possibly some cardiac arrhythmias.[5]

I felt that concentrated sodium citrate (23%) could greatly diminish the incidence of CRBSI in dialysis patients, improve their health and well-being, and save the cost and stress of catheter removal and replacements. I knew that the product would be safe in general use, as long as instructions were followed and common sense prevailed.

I contacted MedComp, the company that was marketing the Ash Split Cath catheter[2], about the market need for our new catheter lock. Their president Tony Madison understood the problem of CRBSI, was very enthusiastic about the idea, and decided to license the product and its pending patents from us. The only form of sodium citrate for intravenous (IV) use available in a small bottle in the U.S. was 47%. The other sodium citrate for IV use was 4% concentration and came in large bags. Developing and obtaining FDA approval for a catheter lock specific for dialysis catheters would be a long and expensive project. Tony's resolution was to place bottles of 47% citrate into kits containing the Split-Cath catheter. I had some misgivings about this step because the bottles contained 30 ml of solution, much more than needed for one catheter placement. I did check to make sure that our packaged Instructions for Use indicated that catheters should be locked with ONLY the catheter volume marked on the catheter extension sets, and that the citrate should be diluted before use. Further the 47% bottle of sodium citrate was clearly marked that it MUST be diluted before use. Our safety analysis indicated a wide margin of safety for a 23% lock solution, even if injected at many times the catheter volume.

In 2007, the worst happened. MedComp received a call from the FDA regarding a mishap in Illinois. It seems that a surgeon had finished placing a CVC for dialysis and injected 10 ml of 47% sodium citrate straight through one lumen of the catheter. The patient immediately had a cardiac arrhythmia and was resuscitated but died several days later. In the telephone conversation, the FDA pointed out that this was an off-label use of sodium citrate as a catheter lock, and that the product was not currently registered with the FDA (though it had been on the market for a long time). FDA asked MedComp to stop supplying sodium citrate for any use. In a few days, FDA published a warning that concentrated sodium citrate was to be used ONLY for white cell isolation during cytopheresis procedures.[81] MedComp removed the bottle of sodium citrate from all kits in production and recalled kits with the bottle in them.

We were devastated by this news, of course. The FDA response to this episode was warranted, but it seemed to me to done without any consideration of the po- tential benefits of the product. Every year over 5000 patients on hemodialysis die due to CRBSI. Here for the first time was a catheter lock solution that could serve as an effective anticoagulant for the catheter AND minimize the risk of CRBSI. And because one physician grossly misused the product, against written instructions, concentrated sodium citrate was to be prohibited from use as a catheter lock in the USA.

Another and larger irony was soon apparent. Because our laboratory was the first to demonstrate that concentrated sodium citrate was antibacterial, we were able to obtain patents covering this use of sodium citrate lock solution in the U.S. and in Europe (through the European Patent Office, EPO). In the US the patent was active, but of course we had no marketable product. In Europe, after the patent was approved it was "contested" in a court in the Netherlands in a case brought by the Dutch company Dirinco. They argued that since sodium citrate has been known for centuries, and since it is known to function as an anticoagulant, its use as a catheter lock solution was obvious. Dirinco lost the case, then lost an appeal. In a final appeal to a magistrate judge for the EPO, their case was APPROVED. So, in the U.S. we had an active patent but no product. In all of Europe, we had at that time a very popular product and to this day, 10%, 30% and 47% citrate are widely used as catheter lock. These sodium citrate catheter locks have been shown to greatly diminish the rate of CRBSI in patients with dialysis catheters.[82,83,84] But we have no patent coverage and therefore, no royalties.

LESSONS LEARNED:

A. In developing a product, make every effort in the original publication and the packaging to stress the importance of following standard procedures in its use. Do not count on physicians reading the enclosed Instructions for Use or even the labels on the bottles.

B. In licensing a product to a major company, find out which components the licensee plans to purchase and from whom. Ask whether the components have been properly registered with the FDA.

C. When a product is licensed from an inventor or small company to a major company, many factors affect the major company's decisions about what the marketed product will be and how it will be marketed. The costs and potential revenues of various forms of the product will be a major factor. If you feel uneasy about how the product might be used (or mis-used), have long and serious conversations with the licensee, and participate in the choice of options. In the case of concentrated citrate, the expensive and slow course of developing a product specifically for dialysis catheter lock would have been a better course. If this course had been taken, concentrated sodium citrate catheter lock would be on the market today in the U.S, just as it is in Europe and around the world.

D. Even issued patents can be challenged in court, sometimes successfully.

Chapter 9
Zuragen™; A Bridge Too Far?

I   suppose I could have (or should have) given up on catheter locks in general after the concentrated citrate debacle discussed in Chapter 8,[85]but I was continually frustrated and saddened each time I saw a dialysis patient with catheter related blood stream infection (CRBSI). I knew that a catheter lock with 7% sodium citrate con- centration would create a density about equal to blood and keep the lock from falling out of the catheter. It would have better anticoagulant properties than the usual 4% sodium citrate, but would have little antibacterial effect. What was needed was a chemical with antiseptic properties to add to the sodium citrate, but which one? I was walking through the pharmacy at our local hospital one day and saw it sitting on the shelf: a bottle of Methylene Blue! This compound, like most dyes, had antiseptic properties. Methylene blue when given orally is absorbed and excreted by the kidneys, where it is effective as a urinary antiseptic. It is given intravenously to provide
dye in the urine to mark ureters during surgery and to treat methemoglobinemia.

So I asked our biochemist Janusz Steczko at Ash Access to determine if adding methylene blue to 7% sodium citrate increased the antibacterial efficacy. The results were surprisingly positive. In combination[86] the two chemicals were much more potent than either one alone. In other words, they were synergistic! If we added methyl- paraben and propyl- paraben, standard preservatives used for solutions in multi-use- vials, then all three were synergistic and the mixture was exceedingly powerful in killing bacteria (as shown in Figure 13). They inactivated bacteria within biofilm, and there were no signs of bacteria forming resistance! A further study showed that the mixture not only killed bacteria within S. Aureus biofilm but physically removed the biofilm from plastic surfaces in fifteen minutes.[87] It looked like we had a winner as an antibacterial catheter lock, and one with a low concentration of sodium citrate.

Bob and I realized that to prove benefits of an antibacterial catheter lock in dialysis CVC would require a large clinical trial, prospectively randomized. Dialysis patients with sepsis often do not have classic signs of sepsis such as fever or high white count, but other symptoms such as rigors, chills, confusion, hypotension and tachycardia. Further, defining CRBSI due to CVC for dialysis is difficult. Unlike CVC for infusion, dialysis catheters are not removed and cultured when there are signs of infection, so defining

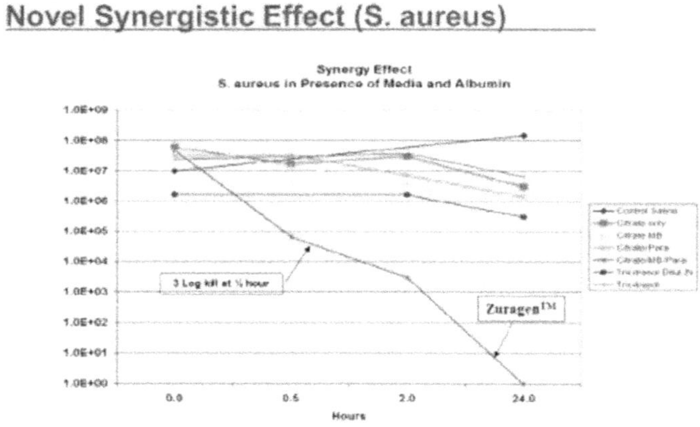

Figure 13. Syngergistic antibacterial effect of sodium citrate, parabens and meth- ylene blue. These were components of the Zuragen™ catheter lock solution.

CRBSI requires concordance of bacterial cultures from blood drawn through the catheter and peripheral blood.

Bob and I discussed how to proceed with this expensive project. Options for funding included raising funds from existing shareholders, using royalty revenue from the Ash Split-Cath, and applying to NIH for an SBIR grant to support the clinical trial (which we eventually received). We decided to go ahead with tests of biocompatibility and toxicity testing. As expected, the animal tests showed no toxicities of any kind.

We wrote up a draft IDE proposal with data collected thus far and sent it to the device division of the FDA (CDRH). We outlined a prospective randomized clinical trial com- paring the incidence of CRBSI in dialysis patients with the citrate-methylene blue- parabens lock (eventually called Zuragen™) versus high concentrations of heparin. The trial would be large (400 patients) and have statistical power to conclusively measure differences in rate of CRBSI. CDRH assured us that they would be the primary reviewer for the lock solution since it did fit the definition of a device (having primarily physical/mechanical action, and functioning within the catheter, not in the bloodstream). They said the Drug division (CDER) would also review the proposal, in a secondary role.

In the next few months we found the CDRH staff to be generally supportive though their review was very thorough and they had asked a number of reasonable questions. They pointed out that there really is no "predicate" device which would support a 510(k) application to the FDA for approval for a catheter lock in CVC for dialysis. They firmly stated that use of a catheter lock in a CVC is "different" from use in a CVC for infusion or a peripheral IV catheter. The only FDA-approved catheter lock solution is very dilute solution of heparin, which is ineffective in maintaining patency in CVC for dialysis. Heparin is widely used for catheter lock in CVC for dialysis at 1000 units/ml or more but this use is entirely off-label. We agreed that the route to market would include a Pre-Market Approval (PMA) with clinical trial, for approval of the catheter lock as a device.

Then we met with staff of CDRH and scientists and physicians from CDER. There really was little agreement between CDRH and CDER on a number of important points. CDER stated that they considered a catheter lock to be a drug if it had any chemical function, whether inside the catheter or not. One staff member said "since methylene blue is a drug, Zuragen™ is a drug!" There was no agreement on the definition of CRBSI dialysis catheters. The committee did agree that concordant blood cultures drawn from a catheter lumen and from peripheral blood was the best evidence of CRBSI, without a catheter tip culture. In the draft protocol, we pro- posed that a "peripheral" blood sample could be obtained by drawing a blood sample from the arterial line of the dialyzer system with the blood pump running about 300 ml/min (rather than using a needlestick in a vein). I argued that there is no way that this sample could be different in bacterial count from the peripheral blood. This point was later proven by Dr. Lok, with an elegant study.[88]

The CDRH group asked us to provide objective indications for drawing blood cultures during the study. The most objective and specific indication of an infection was fever, so we did reluctantly define the primary endpoint of the study as CRBSI shown by "concordant bacteria found in both the catheter and peripheral blood...in subjects demonstrating a temperature > 38°C". During the meeting we explained that many patients on dialysis do not have high fevers with CRBSI, since the patients are normally hypothermic. The IDE protocol stated that blood cultures should also be performed if patients had other signs of sepsis such as tachycardia, confusion or hypotension. The protocol included a secondary endpoint analysis of CRBSI based on symptoms other than fever. At the end of the session, one physician member of CDRH spoke positively of the need for an antiseptic catheter lock in hemodialysis patients, but the reception by the rest of the FDA staff was muted. This physician was transferred to another position within the government a couple of weeks later.

The meeting ended cordially, but the tension between CDRH and CDER was palpable. Some months later, after over one year of discussions with the FDA, Bob and I were both tired of the continued struggle with the FDA over the wording of this IDE, and gave in on the primary endpoint. The FDA approved the application. The whole process of IDE approval required more than two years.

To manage the clinical trials, Bob approached Roland Winger, an engineer who had already shown good management skills in working with Bob. Roland was a "by the books" type of leader. The trial was soon launched and progressed well. As expected, there were few adverse events, none related to catheter lock solutions. When the trial was about 1/3 completed Roland told me that we were not getting very many positive blood cultures, from control or treated groups of patients, about half the expected rate. I said something like "it's too late to change the protocol now, just make sure that the centers know to draw blood cultures on anyone with signs of SIRS." During the trial there was one control patient whose catheter migrated out of the skin, and the staff pushed the cuff back under the skin (a real no-no). The catheter was soon re- moved for a documented infection, but the Data Safety Committee decided that the patient should be censored from the study because of "deviation in protocol" even though the reason for catheter migration was probably catheter infection.

The statistician Dr. Phillip Lavin analyzed the results of the trial and found the overall infection rate was much lower than expected in the control group, at 0.6 per 1000 pt-days. Regarding the primary endpoint, patients with temperature > 38oC and concordant blood cultures were less frequent in the Zuragen™ group than the heparin group. However, the results barely missed statistical significance (P=0.055). Had the one patient with a migrated catheter not been removed from the study, the P value would have been less than 0.05. Analyzing patients with CRBSI defined as concordant blood cultures drawn for any cause, the difference in incidence was highly significant between the two populations (Figure 14).[89] Patency of catheters was better maintained with Zuragen™ than with 5000 units of heparin per lumen, 0 catheters lost due to patency failure versus 4 (P=0.04). Serious adverse events and deaths were all higher in the heparin group, though results were not quite significant.

We were enthused about the results of the clinical trial but of course disappointed by the lack of hitting the primary endpoint. A regulatory affairs consultant from DC stated that several devices have been approved to market by the FDA which "missed the primary endpoint" in a clinical trial. CDRH agreed that they would consider approval of a PMA based on our clinical trial data, but they said "It's a long shot." We set up a meeting with the FDA to discuss the proposal.

As we were going through the clinical trial, we talked to a number of major companies regarding their interest in marketing our antiseptic catheter lock. I was approached at a

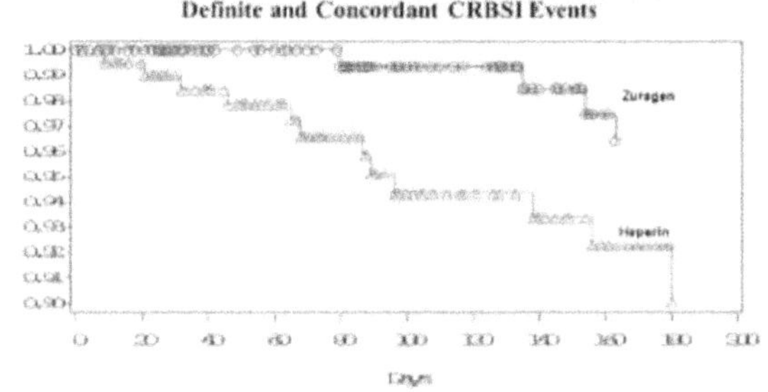

Figure 14. Kaplan-Meier estimates of the cumulative likelihood of freedom from CRBSI in patients with catheter locks of Zuragen™ versus Heparin. The definition of CRBSI was concordant blood cultures from peripheral blood and the catheter. 'Definite" patients had fever at time of drawing blood cultures.

meeting of the ASN by Dr. Jeff Sands and Dr. Jose Diaz-Buxo of Fresenius Medical Care (FMC). They asked "How is it going with the Zuragen™ trial?" They felt that Zuragen™ had a high probability of FDA approval, given results of the trial. A li- cense agreement evolved in which FMC would provide an up-front payment of $4M to Ash Access to offset some costs of Zuragen™ development to date. With FDA approval of Zuragen™ to market for CVC for dialysis, we would receive an additional $16 M in payment. This sounded like a lot, but at this time our estimate of total costs of the product development and clinical trial was $15 M! We were encouraged by the support of FMC, and felt they could help us with the FDA. Plus, we needed the funding to continue our quest for approval of Zuragen™.

We set up a final meeting to discuss our PMA application for approval of Zuragen™. Roland did a great job of presenting our application, starting with the admission that the clinical trial "did not meet the primary endpoint" but showed that by a very strict definition for CRBSI, Zuragen™ significantly decreased the incidence of CRBSI in dialysis patients (Figure 14). The CDER group dismissed the study completely as "missing the primary endpoint." They stated again that "methylene blue is a drug so Zuragen™ is a drug!" After the meeting Dr. Carolyn Neuland from CDRH told me "It wouldn't have mattered if your study had met the primary end- point or not. Zuragen™ would need a second trial because it is a drug." I told her "we can't afford another clinical trial."

We were devastated by this decision, and heavily in debt. The State of Indiana had loaned us two million dollars to help in costs of this trial, and we would have to pay them back eventually with interest. Drs. Sands and Diaz-Buxo were irritated and felt we hadn't told them of all the FDA informal comments in the past. To our amazement, FMC decided not to appeal the decision on Zuragen™ to the Physician Panel. They had "other matters" in discussion with the FDA and did not wish to "muddy the waters." We wrote up a PMA asking for approval of Zuragen™ with indication for patency maintenance of CVC in dialysis, with efficacy equal to he- parin. The FDA pointed out that the trial was not designed to prove this point, and the application would not be approved. We appealed to the Ombudsman, who responded but did not reverse the FDA position.

FMC was also having significant problems in production of vials of Zuragen™. Their contract producer found that the methylene blue in Zuragen™ stained the glass and plastic in their continuous-flow production lines, so Zuragen™ production would require a dedicated line. FMC indicated that they would not pursue Zuragen™ further. Though the product would have had a considerable market in foreign coun- tries, and we had patent coverage in many, they decided that without the FDA approval, pursuing CE mark would be difficult. They cancelled the program and we received none of the expected $16M payment.

It took about two years for FMC to return the right to market Zuragen™ to Ash Access. By this time, licensing of the product to another company was impossible. We decided to license Zuragen™, along with another application of the technology (antiseptic skin preparations solutions) to Zurex Pharma, a spin-off from Ash Access. That product has been FDA-approved to market as discussed in Chapter 10 and Zurex is focusing on this product. I have tried not to think about the problem of CRBSI in dialysis patients for a while, but many physicians keep asking me "What happened to Zuragen™?"

LESSONS LEARNED:
    A. Revolutionary products like Zuragen™ are harder to license to major companies than evolutionary products like the Ash Split Cath.
    B. Licensing a new product to companies is much easier when there is clinical trial data showing safety and efficacy.
    C. However, clinical trials done properly are very expensive, often beyond the budget of small companies such as Ash Access. If at all possible, find a major company to be a partner in funding and managing the clinical trials.
    D. A major company when faced with a regulatory and production pathway that is going to be longer and more expensive than first estimated is quite

likely to cancel the project.

E. Never underestimate the importance of the "primary endpoint" of a clinical trial. Missing the endpoint makes refusal easy for the FDA, even if secondary endpoint analysis already defined demonstrates great benefit of the therapy.

F. Do not expect consistency from the FDA, especially between the drug and device divisions.

G. In the trial, we assured that nurses adhered to best practices in handling CVC for dialysis. As a result, the rate of CRBSI fell dramatically in the control group with heparin catheter locks. The "Hawthorne Effect" is real.

Chapter 10

ZuraGard™: Being second with a better product

In the course of developing the catheter lock Zuragen™, we realized that another potential use of the citrate-parabens-methylene blue solution would be an anti- septic skin cleanser for preparation of patients for surgery,[90,91,92] My experience in placement of tunneled central venous catheters (CVC) for dialysis convinced me that the best way to avoid early infections was to use meticulous aseptic procedures during the placement procedure. This involved cleansing the skin vigorously with a sponge and antiseptic solution, and then draping the surgical site leaving an opening as small as possible around the incision area. It was important to use an antiseptic solution with the greatest early kill of bacteria and longest persistent action. For many years the choice was between chlorhexidine/alcohol (such as ChloraPrep™) and povidone-iodine (such as Betadine®). Chlorhexidine/alcohol had a quicker bacterial kill and more persistent antibacterial effect than povidone-iodine and it captured almost the entire market for pre-surgical "skin prep." ChloraPrep is used in hemodialysis patients as a skin prep before placing a CVC, and before needle sticks into a fistula or graft. However, chlorhexidine/alcohol has some significant problems
and limitations.[93,94,9596]

- There is a significant rebound in growth of bacteria on skin, over forty-eight hours after the skin is prepped with chlorhexidine/alcohol.
- Chlorhexidine/alcohol is somewhat irritating to the skin, which is more apparent when it is used repeatedly and frequently on the same skin area, as in dialysis patients
- Some patients are truly allergic to chlorhexidine, and have immediate skin irritation. Some few have anaphylaxis.
- Increasing numbers of publications are describing bacterial resistance to chlorhexidine.

67

- Chlorhexidine/alcohol is a flammable mixture, due to the inclusion of 70% isopropyl alcohol (IPA). Its use contributes to operative room fires which occur over 200 times yearly in the U.S.. Chlorhexidine/alcohol must be shipped and stored as a hazardous substance.
- Solutions containing alcohol can degrade catheter materials such as polyurethane and silicone , so other somewhat weaker antiseptics are

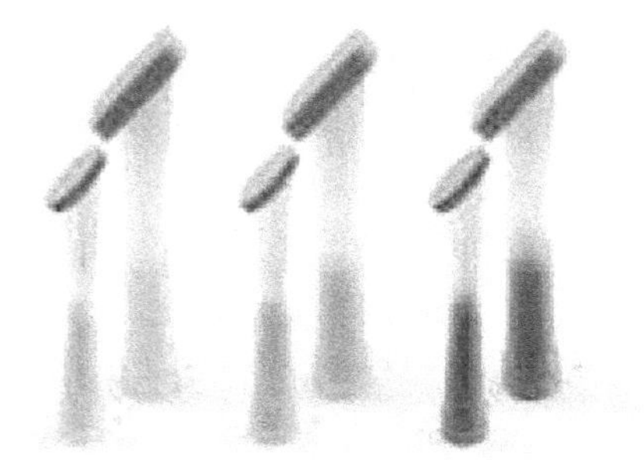

Figure 15. Disposable applicators filled with Zura- Gard™ antiseptic solution, in various colors.

used for cleaning catheter exit sites such as electrolytic chloroxidizer (Amuchina™) or solutions of saline.

It seemed to us that the components of Zuragen™ catheter lock (sodium citrate, methylene blue and parabens) should have the same synergistic antibacterial function against bacteria on the skin surface as they did against planktonic bacteria and biofilm on plastic surfaces. We performed in vitro studies using a skin model, which showed significant antibacterial effects of the Zuragen components, especially when added to the antibacterial effects of alcohol.[92] The tests showed that the solution also had significant antibacterial effects with concentration of alcohol as low as 30%, which would be a solution that is essentially non-flammable.

So, we decided to try to make something out of all the work we'd done on antiseptic solutions. We decided to form (you guessed it) a spin-off company dedicated to the cit- rate-based antiseptic skin preparation. Carmine Durham, a marketing expert had worked closely with Ash Access to find a licensee for Zuragen™ catheter lock. Carmine agreed to be CEO of the new company, but wished the company to be located near his home in Madison, Wisconsin. Wisconsin was encouraging entrepreneurship at that time and several venture capital funds had strong ties to the state. Zurex Pharma was formed and my business partner Bob Truitt became a board member. Ash Access received minority ownership in the new company in exchange for full rights to patents on the antiseptic skin preparation and Zuragen™ catheter lock solution. The first focus of the company was the further development and marketing of the surgical scrub (called ZuraGard™), and a later focus would be on the catheter lock (which they called ZuraSept™).

Things moved along pretty well with the new company. Some highly skilled and dedicated employees began plans for production of the skin prep solution, design of applicators, and clinical testing. Through contract manufacturers, ZuraGard solution suitable for clinical trials was successfully created. Extensive testing confirmed remarkable antibacterial potency of the product. The solution contained 70% isopropyl alcohol, to maintain similarity to ChloraPrep, but also because the potency of 70% alcohol is so high in killing bacteria that it was considered the single active ingredient. The other excipient components were defined: citric acid, alkyl para- hydroxybenzoates and methylene blue (as a colorant). The design of an applicator with a plastic reservoir for the solution was completed and patented (Figure 15).[97]

Though antiseptic skin preparation solutions are considered drugs by the FDA, there are some clearly defined steps in the regulatory process. The animal testing to show safety and biocompatibility of the products is fairly standardized. A clinical trial protocol for testing to diminish skin bacteria on normal volunteers is clearly defined, though techniques are cumbersome and large numbers of subjects are re- quired to assure that allergic reactions are very infrequent. However, when Zurex Pharma submitted a pre-IND to the FDA in 2008, the FDA asked a number of questions which were almost impossible to answer. They wanted to know exactly how much methylene blue might be absorbed through the skin, and whether it would cause any systemic effects. They wanted to know exactly what the interactions were between all of the components of ZuraGard, and whether any components had an active role in the antibacterial function besides alcohol.

Due to the patience and care of those at Zurex Pharma, the FDA questions were answered. Animal trials included plasma tests that showed no absorption of the methylene blue. In vitro testing showed that the 70% IPA was the only active ingredient of ZuraGard. Compared to 70% IPA the other components of ZuraGard made an insignificant contribution to the antibacterial functions, so they were considered excipients and col- orants. The FDA gave approval of an IND protocol to compare the antibacterial function of ZuraGard, ChloraPrep, and control solutions. The FDA required that the tests be per- formed in multiple investigational sites, by two separate testing laboratories. The standard procedures required volunteers not to bathe for some days in order to have sufficient bacterial concentration on skin in the abdominal and inguinal areas. Procedures included vigorous rubbing of the skin preparation solutions onto small portions of skin, and culturing the sites carefully ten minutes and six hours after the skin prep.

Eventually two separate Phase 3 clinical trials were completed, each with hundreds of normal volunteers. The results showed that ZuraGard and ChloraPrep were both effective in diminishing bacterial content on the skin, but with a strong trend towards greater efficacy of ZuraGard™.[98] Later, a meta-analysis was published showing a significant benefit to ZuraGard versus ChloraPrep in bacterial kill.[99] In 2019 the FDA approved ZuraGard™ for the indication "Preoperative skin preparation solution for use in presurgical settings as an antiseptic/antimicrobial agent to reduce bacteria that potentially can cause skin infection."

The company and board turned attention to plans for production of the Zura- Gard™ product, including the applicator with integral solutions of ZuraGard™ (Figure 15). Partly because of the complexity of the newly designed plastic applicator (including no glass components) automated production was more complicated than originally expected. This caused a considerable delay in the marketing studies and the launch of the product. A Beta-site test was the first marketing step, where the product was evaluated by people actually using it in the surgical suite. After all, the product would be used in surgical suites. However, the beta-site testing could not be done until the actual, final product was obtained. The companies interested in investing in or acquiring Zurex Pharma could not make a very high assessment of value without proven production capability and user feedback.

In spite of remarkable success of the company in raising funds, performing pre- clinical studies and accomplishing clinical trials, the board decided a management change was needed in order to speed production of the product. They decided, reluctantly, that Carmine Durham would be replaced as CEO by Paul Vajgrt. Paul has extensive experience in production techniques and in leading new medical technology companies to market success.

Currently, the beta-site trial and a study of surgical site Infection rates are ongoing in a Medical College. Production problems have been solved, and automated steps are minimizing the time and cost of production. Marketing and financing plans are falling in place, and the product in several colors and sizes will be launched sometime in late 2022 or early 2023. Our expectation is that ZuraGard™ will be a highly successful product in the market. Maybe then the company will focus on producing an antithrombotic and antiseptic catheter lock solution.

LESSONS LEARNED:

A. Inventors focus on applying or inventing novel technology to the solution of a significant problem. When the technology is proven to work, especially in clinical trials, the project seems like it is done, from their stand- point. Issues of how to manufacture the final product are left to the licensee, and seem less important than the lab science. They are not. Several critical steps on the way to market success are not possible until the product is available in the final form including: testing in real-world set- tings (beta-site), marketing studies, manufacturing scale-up, marketing campaign, and sales training.

B. The management of a small company to take new technology from bench-top to final product is a tedious and stressful job, requiring lots of patience and perseverance by all involved. A CEO leading a small company from start-up to FDA approval of a new product may not be the best to lead it through production and marketing challenges.

C. Company focus is needed in the process of getting their first product to market. A second product or application of the new technology may be very important and attractive, but devoting limited resources to the second project may be yielding to a siren's song.

D. In a market that is almost entirely filled with a single product (like surgical skin prep), but in which that product is less than perfect, there's plenty of room and some enthusiasm for a new and potentially better product. It's natural to wish to be first on the market with a new type of product. It's sometimes more rewarding to be second, with a better product.

Chapter 11
7% sodium citrate (with benzyl alcohol): "It's difficult to make predictions, especially about the future"[100]

After our publication in 2000 on the antibacterial function of concentrated sodium citrate and its success as a catheter lock for central venous catheters (CVC) for dialysis, concentrated sodium citrate was marketed in Europe and else- where in concentrations of 10%, 30% and 47%.[101] However, due to misuse of concentrated sodium citrate as catheter lock in one patient, the FDA banned highly concentrated citrate as a catheter lock in the US.[102] Numerous published articles demonstrated effective maintenance of patency and diminution of catheter-related bloodstream infection (CRBSI) using concentrated citrate.[103] In 2008 Dr. John Moran and I wrote a position paper on behalf of the American Society for Diagnostic and Interventional Nephrology (ASDIN) indicating the numerous problems of using high concentrations of heparin as catheter lock in CVC for dialysis:[104]

- Systemic anticoagulation
- Induction of anti-heparin antibodies with risk of Heparin-Induced Thrombocytopenia (HIT)
- Inability to prevent bacterial biofilm from forming
- Incompatibility with various antibiotics, when preparing antibiotic catheter lock solutions

The same paper showed advantages of 4% sodium citrate as a catheter lock, with a summary of studies showing that it provides at least as effective maintenance of catheter patency as 1000 units/ml heparin. Other publications followed showing ad- vantages of using this low concentration of sodium citrate over heparin as a catheter lock. [105,106] However, 4% sodium citrate has almost no antibacterial function on its own. In 2012 Dr. Moran and others published a paper showing that gentamicin in 4% citrate was effective in diminishing the rate of (CRBSI) in hemodialysis patients with CVC. [107] Many studies have demonstrated that prophylactic use of antibiotic-containing catheter locks can reduce the incidence of CRBSI in dialysis patients with CVC, but the possibility of inducing antibiotic-resistant bacterial strains is a small but real risk.[103]

We learned from early experience with concentrated citrate lock that it tended to fall out of catheters during instillation especially if the patients were in sitting position.[85] Studies in our laboratory showed that this was because the high concentration citrate locks had a higher density than the blood. This importance of having density of lock solution near that of blood was confirmed by studies of Dr. Hans Polaschegg.[108] We determined that 7% sodium citrate had a density close to the blood of dialysis patients. Addition of various antiseptic agents to the sodium citrate resulted in a solution with high antibacterial and anticoagulant function. Eventually a large randomized clinical trial of the catheter lock Zuragen™ (7% sodium citrate, parabens and methylene blue) showed a marked diminution in incidence of CRBSI in dialysis patients and improved maintenance of patency versus high concentrations of heparin.[109] However, the FDA denied approval to market Zuragen because the study "missed the primary endpoint" of CRBSI in patients and also fever, and be- cause "methylene blue is a drug, not a device."[110] As a result of the FDA decision, support for the project was cancelled by our industry partner, and our company had a significant loss of money on the project.

So in spite of all of our efforts, neither concentrated citrate or Zuragen ever appeared in the US market and we had not provided any new options for catheter locks in the U.S.. Catheter locks of 1000 unit/ml heparin and 4% sodium citrate were still being used off-label and had almost no antibacterial function. I wondered what type of improved catheter lock solution for dialysis could be brought to market? A lock with 7% sodium citrate would be a modest change from the usual 4% concentration, and could be marketed merely for the indication of maintaining catheter patency. Benzyl alcohol was already being used as a preservative in multiple-use vials of 4% sodium citrate to eliminate contaminating bacteria that might enter the bottle during puncture or the syringe and during transfer to the catheter hub. However, in many centers 4% sodium citrate is supplied in pre-filled syringes, a sterile fluid without preservative, and at very high cost.

In 2015, I talked to Bob about whether Ash Access could pursue a third catheter lock, this one much simpler in design than Zuragen™, and with an indication to merely maintain catheter patency. The lock would be 7% sodium citrate with 1.5% benzyl alcohol as preservative. Bob said that we didn't have the resources to conduct even a relatively simple clinical trial on a catheter lock. Further, a catheter lock designed to replace heparin as the standard catheter lock in dialysis would have to be very inexpensive, since it would fall within coverage of the "bundle," a pre-set payment for each dialysis procedure. There might not be enough profit in the product to warrant any company spending a significant amount of money on a clinical trial to obtain FDA approval. So, finding a licensee might be difficult. I nodded my head in agreement, since all of Bob's points were sound.

So of course, I decided to pursue the project anyway. I performed some lab work and found that benzyl alcohol went into solution with sodium citrate quite easily. I arranged for bacteriologic studies at Purdue University which demonstrated that the antibacterial function of the 7% sodium citrate/benzyl alcohol solution was very high, even with several dilutions of the solution. I wrote a clinical trial protocol which utilized a simpler definition of catheter patency than the Zuragen™ trial, and in which all data could be derived from that already being collected in the chair- side computer systems in dialysis units. Although still skeptical, Bob was gracious enough to cover the costs of the lab work, statistical analysis of necessary trial size, and a patent application on the citrate/benzyl alcohol combination, all from the mea ger resources of Ash Access.

We finalized a protocol for the clinical trial and submitted it to the FDA as a pre-IDE. The response letter was gratifying. As long as the primary endpoint of our study was to prove the ability of the citrate solution to maintain catheter patency, and the indication was the same, then the lock solution could be evaluated as a de- vice, not a drug. The FDA made some good suggestions on details of the protocol, which we accepted. They raised a number of questions of course, but these were all answered with some more in vitro work. There were no major concerns about safety of the lock solution since the sodium citrate concentration was only 7%.

Compounding pharmacies supply much of the 4% sodium citrate solutions used for catheter lock in the medical market. I didn't know much about the whole "503(b)" process, but I learned that one of the largest of these companies was Nephron Pharmaceuticals, in Columbia, South Carolina. I decided to call their Pres- ident, Bill Kennedy. I explained to Bill the value of changing the concentration of sodium citrate in the catheter to 7% and of including benzyl alcohol even if the lock was packaged for single-patient use. With a fairly simple clinical trial to show whether 7% sodium citrate maintained catheter patency as well as heparin, the FDA might approve this catheter lock solution for general use in locking CVC for dialysis.

There was a slight pause, and then what Bill said surprised me. He said that as a compounding, outsourcing pharmacy, they make many drugs for many different customers, but he always wanted Nephron Pharmaceuticals to bring its own product to market someday. He explained that compounding pharmacies have considerable leeway for variation in composition of the medicinal products they make, as long as each of the

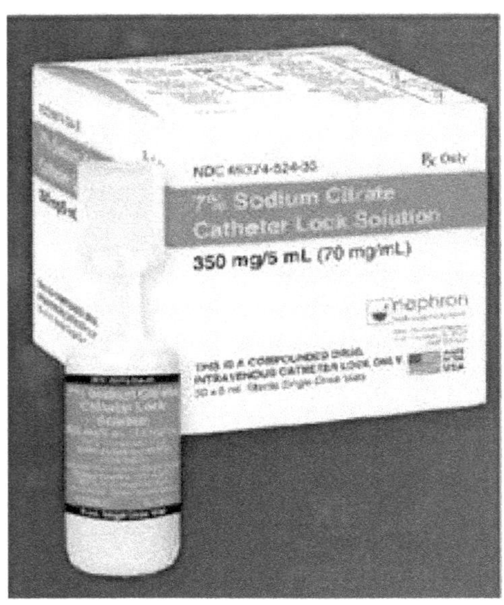

Figure 16. Box label and blow-fill-seal vial of 7% sodium citrate/benzyl alcohol (from Nephron Pharma- ceuticals).

components are already FDA-approved to market. It would be possible for Nephron to produce and supply sodium citrate at 7% concentration as a catheter lock, as long as physicians would order it specifically at this concentration. Adding benzyl alcohol as preservative would be a standard practice. Further, Nephron had just implemented a production line with "blow-fill-seal" technology, in which one automated machine makes small plastic ampoules, fills them with sterile fluid, and adds a frangible seal. When the seal is opened, a female Luer connector is revealed so that a syringe can be directly attached to remove fluid from the ampoule. This would be a perfect pack- age for providing single-patient use of the product.

After a phone-call with Bob Truitt, Bill decided to go forward with a license of the product on a trial basis, allowing the product to be produced and introduced to the mar- ket. We could then obtain some market feedback before making a long-term agreement.

Progress in this project has been as planned, but personnel shortages during the Covid-19 epidemic slowed the production and testing schedule. However, production of this catheter lock was completed in the blow-fill-seal vials, as shown in Figure 16. The product was listed on the nephronpharmaceutical.com website early in 2021. The price for 5 ml vials was significantly less than that for pre-filled syringes of 4% sodium citrate, though somewhat more than the cost of heparin from multi-use vials.

Market response was initially very positive, especially among those who were using 4% sodium citrate for catheter lock in hospitals and dialysis units. Then, curiously, re-orders of the product were low. It was not clear the reasons, but a common response was "we don't see any problems with the 4% sodium citrate we're using currently." Perhaps lingering memories of the FDA warnings about 47% citrate caused hesitation in accepting a very modest increase in concentration, but no one said that. Perhaps all of the commotion of the Covid epidemic interfered with the whole process of physicians evaluating new products. The initial production run had a listed shelf life of six months. When that lot expired, Nephron did not make another production run.

So, what will happen to this somewhat novel lock solution is unclear. Having the lock solution produced and available as a 503(b), special order item would allow a simple study to be done in a few dialysis units, to see if there's an improvement in catheter patency. If a few physicians were willing to submit a protocol to their IRB committees and the proposals were approved, and if Nephron were encouraged to pro- duce the product again, then published results supporting the product would be avail- able. So, perhaps use of the product could expand, and eventually a larger clinical trial might be done to determine whether 7% sodium citrate should be used as a standard catheter lock in dialysis. Even then, what would the market response be? If the cost of the citrate lock solution is slightly higher than the cost of heparin, will a Large Dialysis Organizations (LDO) promote its use? Only if nephrologists actively push their LDO to use 7% sodium citrate as catheter lock solution, instead of heparin.

LESSONS LEARNED:
    A. Choosing the right business partner for developing a new product is essential. The partner must have the right production technology, the right marketing strategy, history with a similar type of product, and a desire to add this type of product to their portfolio. Sometimes finding the right partner requires dozens of contacts. Sometimes only one.
    B. A catheter lock with 7% sodium citrate is an evolutionary step from locks containing 4% sodium citrate. The lock will remain within catheters better and diminish catheter thrombosis. With benzyl alcohol, perhaps it will de-crease incidence CRBSI, perhaps not. Zuragen™ was a revolutionary product, with antiseptic properties to help prevent CRSBI. Evolutionary products should be much easier to bring to market, but it's still not easy.
    C. The downside of evolutionary products is that users do not expect to pay

much more for them than the old, unimproved product. If production and regulatory costs of the product change are significant, and they can't be recovered through higher price of the product, then the product may not be worth pursuing by the licensee company regardless of its apparent benefits. The "bundle" formula for payment of hemodialysis procedures actually inhibits innovation in the dialysis components and procedures.

D. If in my quest to improve catheter locks I had begun with a more modest goal, slightly increasing sodium citrate concentration and adding a preservative, then 7% sodium citrate would probably be the standard catheter lock in dialysis units today. That might have been a smarter move, but obtaining funding and generating enthusiasm would have been more difficult.

Chapter 12
Oral sorbents for small, charged uremic toxins and carbon block for regeneration of dialysate:

My original mission in research was to find a simpler, safer, more convenient way to dialyze patients with ESRD. After the apparent dead-end path of the Allient™ sorbent-based dialysis machine, I realized that regenerating dialysate with a column of sorbents actually does have limitations. [III] The charcoal layer of the Sorb™ column of the old Redy™ system worked exceedingly well in binding organic and protein-bound toxins of kidney failure in dialysate. However, to bind potassium, urea and phosphate and provide bicarbonate the column includes urease, cation exchangers and anion ex- changers. There are a number of problems in a Sorb™ column because of these three layers: variable ammonium capacity, need to monitor ammonium release, release of hydrogen and sodium to dialysate, complete removal of calcium and magnesium from the dialysate, and generation of CO_2 bubbles. With a sorbent column like in the Redy™ system the net transfer of sodium and bicarbonate is predictable, but concentrations in dialysate will vary widely during the treatment. Perfusing the column requires high pressures, and the column expands during dialysis, making UF control difficult. The column itself is heavy, somewhat costly, and is discarded with each treatment.

Thinking of all of these problems made me understand why FMC failed in their redesign of the Allient™ machine. They tried to make it work just like any other dialysis machine. What surprised me more was that four companies creating highly portable dialysis systems currently are using a sorbent column to regenerate dialysate, with the same basic components as the Redy™ Sorb™ column. Fairly complex systems are being implemented to control the individual ion concentrations in dialysate.

In the late 1970s we studied intestinal sorbent binding of various uremic toxins in animal models.[50,65] Through an inlet ostomy we infused large amounts of a mixture of a cation exchanger, calcium carbonate (for phosphate binding), powdered charcoal and urease. In normal rats and goats, the intestinal sorbents were very effective in removing potassium and phosphate, and there was a significant removal of urea (equal to function of approximately one kidney). In anephric animals the urea and phosphate actually stabilized and potassium often decreased below normal.

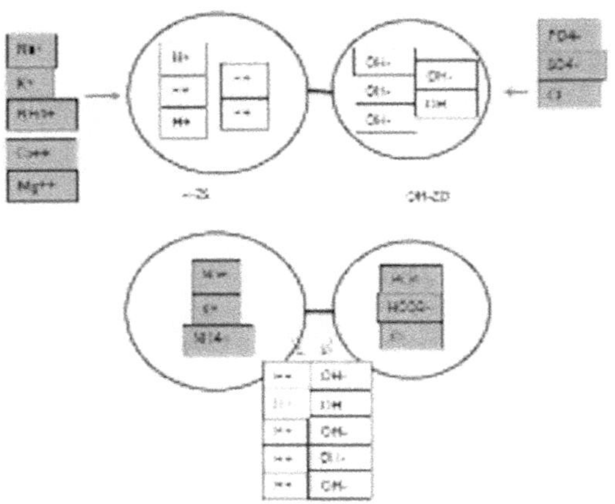

Figure 17: Mixed ion exchanger system with hydrogen-loaded cation exchanger and hydroxide-loaded anion exchanger, a potential oral sorbent for uremic toxins.

However, creatinine clearance was nearly zero, since creatinine (and most other organic toxins) do not permeate the intestinal mucosa very well. I thought that if we had a powerful enough sorbent and administered it orally we could effectively remove five Small and Charged Uremic Toxins (SCUT) from the gut: potassium, phosphate, sodium, hydrogen and ammonium (from urea by urease of bacteria). I decided to make a suspension of hydrogen-loaded cation exchanger with hydroxide-loaded anion exchanger and see if it would remove all of our target small toxins as shown in Figure 17.[112] Since the released hydrogen and hydroxide combine to form water, they disappear from the solution and there are no other counterions. This is the concept of the "mixed bed deionizer" columns used to produce highly purified water.

We chose zirconium phosphate (ZP) as the cation exchanger, which is non-selective and amorphous, and zirconium oxide (ZO) as the anion exchanger, also non- selective and amorphous because these were used in the Sorb columns. In solutions simulating the concentration of ions in small intestine and colon and containing calcium and magnesium, the suspension removed the various toxins exceedingly well, far better than the cation and anion exchangers when used individually. Of course, there was removal of calcium and magnesium from the solutions but capacities for toxin binding remained high.

The first animal trials of this mixture were performed by measuring changes in daily urinary and fecal excretion in as a measure of binding of SCUT in the gut. The sorbents were given by gavage injection, daily. These trials in rats demonstrated complete safety of the mixture at moderately high dosages (2 gm/kilo/day for the sorbent mixture) but very little removal of the target toxins. The trials were sponsored by a major dialysis supply company, but efficacy results were so negative that they dropped out of the project. What were the causes of failure of the ZP/ZO mixture? We thought that the affinity of ZP for divalent cations might have been the problem after all within the gut, or maybe protein, lipids and starches in the gut covered the active sites of the amorphous sorbents, making them inactive.

So, we decided to use sodium zirconium cyclosilicate (SZC, ZS, or Lokelma®) as the cation exchanger in our mixture. This had been developed by Union Carbide and Universal Oil Products (UOP) in cooperation with HemoCleanse as described in a previous chapter.[113] SZC is a synthetic crystal cation exchanger with its active sites inside thin parallel plates. The sites of SZC are selective for monovalent cations over divalent cations, so binding of calcium and magnesium is near zero. Clinical trials and clinical experience have shown that SZC is a remarkably effective oral sorbent for

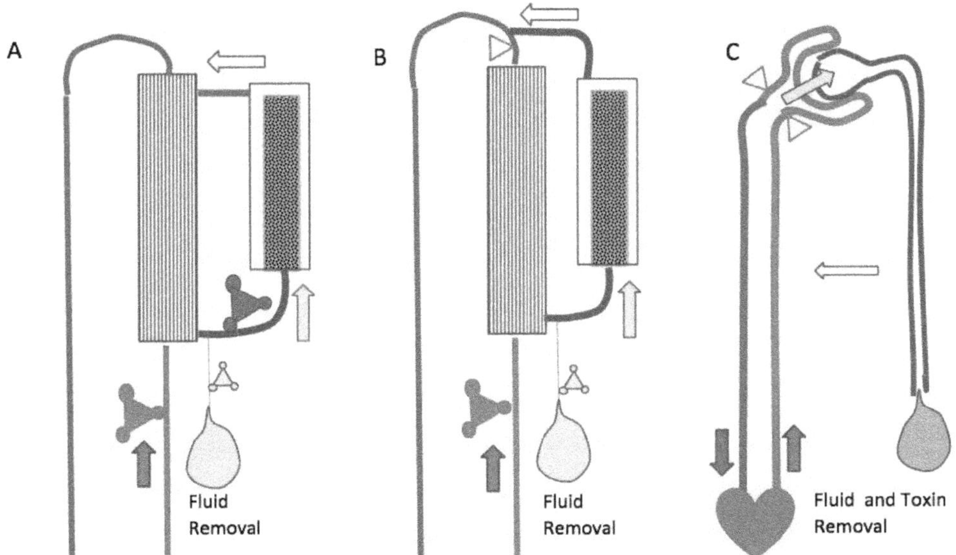

Figure 18. Dialysis circuit with a carbon block cartridge in position on the outflow line of the dialyzer
    A. Schematic of hemodialysis system including a dialyzer, carbon block, blood pump (red), dialysate pump (blue) and pump for removing excess fluid (yellow). Toxin-laden dialysate (yellow arrow) perfuses the carbon block and returns to the dialyzer free of organic toxins (clear arrow). Excess fluid and salt are removed by the ultrafiltrate pump.
    B. Schematic of hemofiltration system including a high permeability dialyzer, carbon block, blood pump (red) and pump for removing excess fluid (yellow). A constriction on the effluent blood line controls the rate of filtration by the dialyzer (clear triangle). Purified filtrate returns directly to the blood (clear arrow).
    C. Schematic of the archetype, the human kidney. Blood flows into the glomerular capillaries (red), which pass a toxin-laden filtrate into the tubules. The tubules absorb the water, salt, and vital chemicals from the filtrate and return it to the blood (clear arrow). The rate of glomerular filtration is controlled by varying constriction of the inflow and outflow capillaries (clear triangles). Excess body fluid exits the tubules and is excreted as urine.

potassium in many types of patients.[114,115,116] So we tested the ZS/ZO in the simulated gut solutions and it worked fine. The sorbent mixture was given by gavage injection again in a study of normal rats. Amazingly, these trials also showed very little removal of the SCUT compounds with exception of phosphate, which was very effective.

I then decided to review all of the animal trials performed by HemoCleanse and also ZS Pharma. This wasn't an easy project because I had been actively involved in only the first very preliminary study. I discovered that if the sorbent mixture was given by gavage injection it had almost no binding of potassium or any uremic toxins in the gut. However, it worked remarkably well if given as a mixture with food. The reason for this difference was not clear, but may have been due to rapid transit of the sorbent through small bowel, induced by gavage injection. So, we performed another animal trial, mixing sorbents with either ZP or ZS into the powdered food given the rats. This trial showed excellent removal of phosphate by the sorbents but little removal of potassium or ammonium. Apparently, some chemical or substance in the gut, in combination with the anion exchanger, is inactivating binding of cations by ZP and ZS. So, we are now planning to test giving the sorbent components at separate times of day, separating the administration of ZP and ZS from the ZO. We are also developing a gas-permeable coating for ZP which will allow ammonium to be removed but prevent direct interaction with gut components, chemicals and other sorbents. We'll see what happens!

In parallel to our oral sorbent project, HemoCleanse maintained an active pro-gram to develop carbon block technology for regeneration of dialysate, mostly through the efforts of Mr. Tom Sullivan, a skilled engineer and scientist.[117] If the oral sorbent worked for SCUT compounds, a very simple dialysis machine could be designed to regenerate dialysate or ultrafiltrate by removing organic toxins, and to remove a small amount of fluid and sodium daily as shown in Figure 18a.

Carbon columns as used in the Sorb™ column were highly effective for removal of small and large m.w. organic toxins but they were not perfect. Typical of carbon columns of that day, they were created with granular particles of activated charcoal, 0.5-2 mm diameter. There were a number of problems with these types of columns, including settling during storage, irregular perfusion, fragility of the carbon and a Lack of capacity for larger organic toxins.

About 1990 Dr. Koslow developed a process by which plastic materials containing a high percentage of powdered activated carbon could be extruded into a porous solid cylinder. The resulting "carbon block" column could then be perfused with liquids from a central lumen to the outside, and the carbon removed impurities from the liquid. Although the spicules of plastic held every particle of the sorbent in place, they did not cover the external active sites of the carbon.[118] This

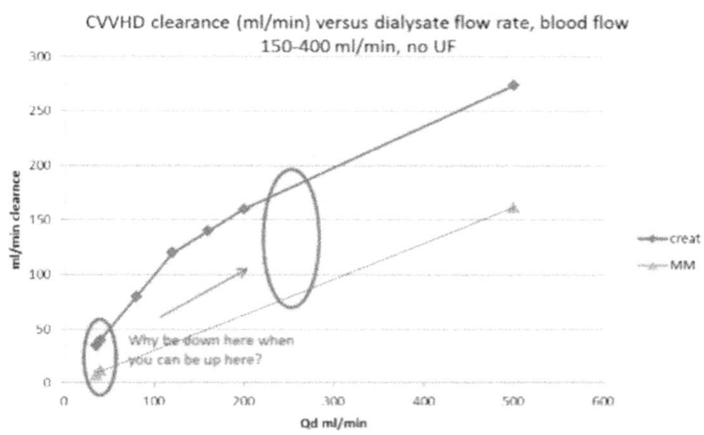

Figure 19..*Relationship of clearance of creatinine and several MMW toxins (aver- aged), versus dialysate flow rate for a CVVHD treatment.*

remarkable invention provided a perfusion column containing powdered charcoal with: a high percentage weight of carbon, modest pressure drops, excellent flow dispersion, very small particle size and almost zero release of fines. Soon, carbon blocks were being used widely as under-the-sink potable water filters, in-line filters for coffee makers, ice machines, and eventually for dialysate water purification.

Tom obtained a variety of carbon blocks from various commercial sources, many of which contained powdered carbon from coconut shells, which was the same source used for the carbon layer of the Sorb™ column and our powdered carbon in Liver Dialysis™. In terms of chemical selectivity and capacity, the specifications for carbon blocks mostly related to function in removing toxins from drinking water, such as removal of volatile organic carbons (VOC), chlorine, and chemicals contributing to taste and odor. There were no specifications for removing organic uremic toxins. Tom set up an elaborate testing bed to determine the efficiency of removal and capacity of various columns for toxins of kidney and liver failure, including creatinine, bilirubin, middle and high molecular weight dyes, etc. Large tanks contained dialysate with high concentrations of a toxin which was perfused through the columns.

We were able to find a few columns on the commercial market with suitable binding characteristics to work in regeneration of dialysate for treatment of kidney failure, liver failure and drug overdose. But every time we found a suitable carbon block, we soon learned that it was not available any more or the company making it was purchased by another company. Further, none of the columns were produced under GMP conditions suited for medical devices.

One day I was ordering a Continuous Veno-Venous Hemofiltration-Dialysis (CVVHD) treatment using a NxStage System 100 dialysis machine for a patient in the ICU. As I ordered the usual dialysate flow of two liters per hour (33 ml/min) from five- liter sterile bags, and a blood flow rate of 300 ml/min, I thought "What a shame!" At this puny dialysate flow rate, the highest clearance of anything would be 33 ml/min, and for large organic toxins much less than that. I realized that if I had our carbon block column I could regenerate the dialysate and greatly increase removal of the important toxins. I went back home and sketched out a way to regenerate dialysate in a CVVHD system, as in Figure 18a. I also calculated the relationship of dialysate flow to middle molecular toxins. As shown in Figure 19, at a dialysate flow rate of 250 ml/min and re- generation of the dialysate by carbon, clearance of middle molecular toxins by CVVHD could increase from about 10 m/min to nearly 100 ml/min. Of course, removal of SCUT and replenishment of bicarbonate would still be controlled by replacing the five-liter bags of dialysate, on a usual schedule or sometimes even less.

So, I envisioned the first use of this carbon block column in regenerating dialysate during CVVHD. We demonstrated that every middle-sized uremic toxin we tested was effectively bound by our best carbon blocks including indole acetic acid, para cresol sulfate, and indoxyl sulfate.[117] Removal of B-2 macroglobulin by carbon had already been shown.[119] One moderate sized carbon block could regenerate CVVHD fluid for twenty four hours or more. We showed that carbon blocks can be sterilized by gamma radiation without loss of any chemical binding properties. In large production volumes, the carbon block cartridge should be relatively inexpensive to produce, certainly less than the cost of two or three bags of sterile dialysate to the hospitals. In many patients, fewer bags of dialysate would be used for CVVHD, since the frequency of changing bags would be adjusted down if the patient had normal or near normal values of urea, potassium, phosphate and hydrogen in the blood.

With this focus for our first application of the carbon block column, I began to search for partners in this project. I approached all three of the companies who marketed CRRT machines in the US. I learned that they would not build any device that diminished sales of sterile dialysate in bags to hospitals. I then approached companies who created and marketed water purification devices for dialysis. They under- stood the device and had the capability to make it, but were not in the business of selling sterile disposables for CRRT.

I next finally turned my attention to companies that were creating anything new in dialysis therapy. By chance I met a nurse/manager from a company called Nephros at an ASN meeting. I had heard of this company because they were the first (and only) company to have obtained approval by the FDA to market an attachment to convert dialysis machines to perform hemodiafiltration (HDF), for better removal of larger molecular weight toxins. For once, our discussion didn't begin with the question "what are middle-molecular toxins?" I met with Daron Evans their CEO and he filled me in on the how the company was making HDF practical. Be- sides this achievement, Nephros had an active business in creating filters to produce sterile fluid for use in pharmaceutical companies, pharmacies and industry. Daron seemed genuinely interested in my project and immediately understood the benefits of the regeneration of sterile fluid in CVVHD. We agreed that the carbon block could be used to remove uremic toxins from the filtrate of a hemofilter, concentrating the toxins within the block (Figure 18 b). This mimics the archetype native kidney, which concentrates toxins in a small volume of urine (Figure 18 c). We agreed to pursue R&D of the carbon block jointly, and we completed a simple license agreement from HemoCleanse to Nephros. The Nephros company has since "spun off" its renal-related technology into a separate entity, Specialty Renal Products (SRP). Although the major focus of SRP has been to redesign their HDF module to make it simpler to use, they have also made progress on the carbon block project. SRP has communicated with the FDA to define the regulatory path for the carbon block column, and helped to define some built-in components like filters. The time course of the project, and even its outcome is still uncertain however.

LESSONS LEARNED:

A. When there are multiple projects that would benefit from developing one device component, do it! A common adage is that "nobody does anything for just one reason." Our research team first used powdered carbon to remove toxins of hepatic failure and drug overdose from dialysate. The goal of simplifying dialysis was conceivable, if we had oral sorbents for SCUT and the carbon block for dialysate regeneration. Then I saw a great application in improving the efficacy of CVVHD.

B. The original reasons for developing a new medical device may evolve to several potential applications by the time you finish the project. That's great!

C. Beware of using components that are commercially available in your new device, especially if they don't fit your needs exactly. These products may be discontinued, renamed, or modified in the future. This was the case with our trying to use carbon blocks made for drinking water purity.

D. In searching for a licensee, learn all you can about all products they make. The breadth of their product production, marketing and interests may surprise you.

SUMMARY and CONCLUSIONS

If frustration is the father of invention, and necessity is the mother, their children are driven by both to write biographies. What can be learned from a review of these twelve projects (drugs and devices) conducted by our small companies? Most projects have had the goal of improving hemodialysis technology so that dialysis could be simpler, safer and better suited for the home environment. Other projects tried to adapt dialysis to treat previously untreatable conditions (such as liver failure and hepatorenal syndrome). Here are the lessons I've learned from the R&D projects above:

A. There are plenty of new ideas and approaches to treatment of ESRD among nephrologists.

Every nephrologist experiences frustration with dialysis in treatment of ESRD. After all, we became physicians because we had empathy, and it is painful and shameful to watch patients suffer adverse symptoms and poor outcomes on our therapy. I imagine every reader has said to himself "there has to be a better way." Those with a solid education in science or engineering and an inventive nature have prob- ably thought of as many new approaches as I have (maybe some better ones).

Contrary to popular opinion (even among those writing articles on dialysis therapy), there were dramatic improvements in dialysis therapy between the 1960s and 1990s:

- Hollow fiber dialyzers provided much greater chemical efficiency and minimized blood volume (compared to coil and flat plate dialyzers)
- High permeability membranes improved clearance of middle molecular weight toxins and phosphate
- Controlled filtration allowed accurate fluid removal at constant rate (versus the ever-changing and inaccurate predictions based on dialyzer Kuf

and transmembrane pressures)
* Bicarbonate dialysate provided natural buffering of the patient, without symptomatic exposure to synthetic bases (like acetate and lactate)
* Central dialysate delivery systems and pre-mixed concentrates eliminated most mistakes in creation of the dialysate (versus the manual creation and alteration of dialysate baths)
* Central blood volume measurement detected whether the patient is tolerating the current ultrafiltration rate (rather than waiting for symptomatic hypotension).
* Arteriovenous fistulas, synthetic grafts and tunneled dialysis catheters provided fairly reliable blood access for many months to years, without the need for invasive procedures at the start of each dialysis (like femoral catheters) or repeated surgeries on arterial vessels (like arteriovenous shunts).
* Ultrasound evaluation of blood vessels and ultrasound guided needle entry has made placement of dialysis access devices safer, more accurate and effective (as opposed to blind sticks and surgical guesses).

Each of these improvements was the result of collaboration of many physicians, scientists and companies. The improvements were welcomed by the nephrology market when they became available, and there was not much market resistance to clearly new and better ideas. The modifications in dialysis procedure allowed dialysis to be performed more efficiently, in shorter time and with fewer adverse symptoms than the older technology. The outpatient "in-center" model for delivering dialysis developed partly because of these technologies. A unit with many patients benefitted from central dialysate delivery systems. More reliable vascular access al- lowed dialysis to be performed without sterile, invasive procedures. Growth of in- center units began when Medicare coverage for dialysis services was implemented in 1973, but expanded greatly in the 1980s and 1990s as the business model continued to be improved. As the "brick and mortar" locations of dialysis expanded, the technology stabilized and innovation in dialysis slowed. Thus, dialysis therapy followed the model of other industries. Widespread implementation of any one technology greatly increases the cost of changes, and thus slows further innovation.

The Kidney Health Initiative was formed in cooperation between the American Society of Nephrology and the FDA in 2012.[120] The stimulus was a "dearth of research and development in nephrology" as evidenced by the fact that there are few randomized and controlled studies published regarding kidney therapies. The KHI hoped to "enable the kidney community as a whole to provide the right drug, device, or biologic for administration to the right patient at the right time..." This is a laud- able goal, but choosing the "right drug" or "right device" is not a stimulus for developing a new drug or a new device. The closest the program has come to fostering true innovation is the KidneyX Phase II prizes, which as discussed below involved widespread competition for only a few sizeable prizes. A better display of innovative new ideas is in the KHI "roadmap" for development of renal replacement therapies developed by Dr. Fokko Wieringa, Murray Sheldon and others, and the IFAO- ASAIO session of 2020 on the Implantable Artificial Kidney.[121,122]

New ideas are available for new approaches in dialysis therapies, such as the Implantable Artificial Kidney. Many of the ideas are well-founded and logical, and should be workable. Turning the ideas to reality is one problem, and convincing nephrologists to learn about new therapies and adopt them into their practice is an even larger challenge. An example is peritoneal dialysis, still vastly under-utilized about four decades since it was perfected.

B. Many good ideas "die on the vine" because the inventors don't have the resources, time or dedication to develop workable prototypes.

I have a number of nephrologists who call me with a new idea to solve a problem in dialysis therapy. Their enthusiasm is obvious as they tell me of their new approach. My first recommendation to them is that they develop a workable prototype and figure out some way to demonstrate its advantages. The prototype doesn't have to be elaborate or even be the proper scale, it just has to work (or in the language of patent attorneys be "reduced to practice"). I can sense the disappointment in some of the callers, when they think of the work and cost of getting to a prototype stage.

Of the twelve projects I reviewed above, every one of them began with a laboratory prototype of some form or other, and some type of testing to prove the physical or chemical principles. The funding of our radical SSRD (#2 above) from Eli Lilly began with a presentation I gave to the Vice President of Eli Lilly. At the dinner table, I unwrapped a prototype of this wearable artificial kidney, sat it on the table and turned it on. As a motor ran on D cell batteries and a bellows went in and out, pink fluid was drawn from a cup, disappeared into membranes in the middle of the black sorbent suspension and came out crystal clear. The removal of chemical dye was predictable and expected, but the impression it left was dramatic (fortunately the thing didn't leak). We got our funding at the Bioengineering lab, and cooperation with Eli Lilly in the project was truly enjoyable. In projects such as development of new catheters, the prototype and some in vitro testing results did most of the convincing of the licensing company.

Of course, just having a prototype is no guarantee of success in funding or in the market. For revolutionary devices with new technology, the first devices to treat a disease (like liver failure), or those where therapy will be done in special settings (like home dialysis), the start-up company may have to carry the project much further down the road before a major company is interested in cooperating. But, a successful prototype serves to boost confidence in the product and in you, your "... colleagues, and early investors.

Learn from the prototype just how well it meets the functional requirements of your invention. Don't become dedicated to any one idea, design or component. No matter how much work has gone into it, if one part is not satisfactory, scrap it. Look for new designs or technology to achieve the needed function.

C. For small companies and inventors, finding the funding to carry project forward is usually the first consideration; however, finding the right corporate partner is equally important.

When an entrepreneurial company is formed, the focus is on the new product or process. The "exit strategy" is usually pretty vague, but usually involves either a license of the technology to a major company (when the technology is proven) or a buy-out of the small company by the larger one (at some later stage). Very few inventors and entrepreneurs really wish to form a company for production and marketing of their newly invented product. With some products such as implantable catheters, setting up efficient production processes as a small company is nearly impossible. Our central venous catheter developments (Ash Split Cath™ and CentrosFLO™) were licensed after being created in prototype form. The companies worked out the final design, production processes, sterilization techniques, packaging, marketing, etc. The same was true for three peritoneal dialysis catheters we've developed (discussed below).

Even for revolutionary products which will require clinical trials to prove efficacy and safety, it is never too early to begin discussion with major companies. After obtaining patent protection, begin communicating with the companies that market products which are the most similar to your product. If it's a savvy company, they already know more about you and your company than you expect. It takes considerable time to convey all that you've learned about the disease you're treating, the market, current technology, how your product works, and what should be the benefits. This is an educational process for the company you're approaching, but also for you. You will learn about the breadth of products of the larger company, the goals and directions, and the decision makers. You will undoubtedly tune up your presentation each time it is re- peated. Contacts within the company can be open lines for news on your progress. Some companies just seem to "fit" with you, your product, and your needs. Find one.

D. Before proceeding to clinical trials, be sure that the device or drug is absolutely as perfect as you can make it.

Every blood treatment system is a complex collection of a number of technologies. Especially for components that have been specially developed for this device, they must be completely tested for reliability and accuracy. In our BioLogic-HD machine (Chapter 3 above) the optical blood flow monitors never worked as well as we had hoped, and ultrasonic flow probes were too expensive for production machines. Though the monitors were merely an alarm system, when they did indicate a problem, we couldn't be sure whether the alarm and data were real or not. Added to all the other problems the home dialysis machine was facing, knowing it needed some redesign didn't help much.

There is great advantage in using components that exist on the market in a new therapy. However, if the product isn't exactly what you need, this is not a short cut. That was the case when we supplied 47% sodium citrate for use as a catheter lock solution, and instructed physicians to dilute it before using. It was also the case when we pursued using carbon block columns designed for drinking water purification, when our application would be in regenerating dialysate. Neither short cut led to market success.

E. Of those ideas which are proven effective and safe in clinical trials, there are still innumerable hurdles between proven success of the device and wide- spread market adoption (the real goal of the inventor and company).

Every step along the way from idea to market success is highly valuable, since risk of the project decreases with each step. However, the road doesn't always smooth out, sometimes it gets rougher as you travel. Of our twelve projects, none failed in the steps of prototyping, patenting, lab testing or clinical trials. Only one failed in animal testing, from an adverse effect we could not have predicted. A failure of FDA approval stopped only one of our projects, a drug-device combination. An unexpected change in government regulations stopped our first home dialysis ma- chine. Dr. Kolff's WAK project and our Allient™ machine project each failed after license to major manufacturing and marketing companies. The companies in each case decided to re-design to become much more like a traditional dialysis machine. Our concentrated citrate lock solution was a market success in Europe, but was taken off the market in the U.S. because one physician badly misused the product.

    F. **The final step towards market success requires that practicing physicians are as frustrated and dissatisfied with current solutions as you are, so that they will want to use the new product.**

When we first use a therapy on a patient and see their immediate improvement, it is a gratifying and sometimes amazing experience. However, as our experience with the therapy increases, we see a few immediate complications, and after some more time, later complications and failure of the therapy. Therefore, not all physicians have the same degree of frustration with dialysis as practiced now. Further, the physicians develop their practice within the boundaries and practices of large dialysis organizations and hospitals. Even if a physician has read about your new improvement in the therapy, and would like to use it, they realize that convincing the LDO or hospital to acquire the product may be an arduous process. Early adopters are those physicians willing to put significant effort into changing local practices. The more revolutionary the product, the harder the work and the more support they need from the sponsoring companies. Most physicians are in the average adopters, who will use the product when available, but will not promote use of it.

We had one product that was well adopted and used by early adopters, the Bio- Logic- DT™ (Liver Dialysis™). The original marketing plan was a "hub and spoke" approach centered on large liver transplant centers and reaching into referring hospitals. The initial marketing was to these centers, each of which had physicians who knew how to choose patients who would benefit most from the machine. Ongoing research projects were focused on careful measurement of patient benefits. When marketing was expanded widely, the machines were not used on optimal patients and research projects were not supported well. The result was a marketing failure.

G. In the medical market, the probability of overall success of a project is greater for products that are evolutionary than those that are revolutionary.

When I was growing up, I always wanted to be first. On the basketball court, my older brother already had that advantage (and also a lot more skill and size). I excelled a bit more in the classroom, but still not having the highest grade on a test bothered me.

Looking over the twelve projects above, there is a trend that appears. Our first forays into dialysis improvements focused on revolutionary changes in the technology and even new device indications. For ESRD patients, it was towards wearable or highly portable machines using sorbents to absorb toxins. For liver failure patients, the sorbents were tuned to treatment of liver failure, a new indication. It was kind of fun being first.

Our greatest market success was however with products that were more evolutionary than revolutionary. Zirconium cyclo-silicate was not the first cation ex- changer to be used as an oral sorbent for potassium. Polystyrene sulfonate held that position for fifty years (Kayexalate™). Patiromer (Veltassa™) was second, and ZS- 9 was third to reach the market. It had some significant advantages, so its use expanded rapidly. Similarly, the Ash Split Cath™ was not the first tunneled dialysis catheter. It was really an improvement on the older single-body Mahurkar catheter. It reached the position of the most popular tunneled dialysis catheter on the market, not too long after introduction.

Over time, the products we have focused on have become more evolutionary than revolutionary. At times I wonder whether we could have started with these types of products. But on the other hand, when the inventor is young and the product has unique technology and exciting potential, enthusiasm in the investment com- munity and company supporters come naturally. Also, it's easier for the inventor to remain enthusiastic when there's a good chance for him to live long enough to see the project completed and see how the market responds.

H. Keep the faith.

Turning to another question, how can we each contribute to artificial organs? I'm seventy-six years old now, so I'm old enough to give advice but also too old to change my ways. Here are ten simple rules for any young physician or researcher, which I described in my Presidential Address to ASAIO in 2006:[123]
* Know the problem
* Know but doubt the paradigm
* Train with the best in scientific method
* Use the newest tools, model all you can
* Focus
* Collaborate
* Communicate, Publish
* Be patient
* Be careful
* Keep balance in your life, strong family ties and faith, but maintain humility.

A word to those bright and young physicians who, like me see problems in their practice, and search for solutions. Good for you. The world needs people just like you. Besides, with your ambition and creativity, you are destined (or doomed) to search for solutions. Most of the technologies and approaches we use in dialysis came from physicians searching for the right technology, just like you and me. But realize that just coming up with the idea is only the start of a long, long commitment that's needed before an invention becomes an innovation. Looking over the above twelve chapters should show that there are numerous ways that any new technology can fail to have market success and really make a difference in patients' lives. Even after the idea is proven, the patent is issued and the FDA approves the product to market, you can see it fade away. Get as much help as you can, as quick as you can, and throughout each stage. But don't give up. You have more time and resilience than you think.

Take a look at our history of device and drug development in Table 1. We had five serious projects to develop a sorbent-based dialysis system suitable for the home or providing effective therapy in new applications. While all were successful technically, none was a market success. The sixth sorbent application was in the oral sorbent therapy of hyperkalemia, and so far Lokelma® has been remarkably successful in therapy of hyperkalemia. The current approach to dialysate regeneration involves use of a carbon block column to regenerate dialysate, which is a highly practical method for removal of the important organic middle molecular toxins. However, its success depends also on our development of an oral sorbent therapy to remove the small and charged uremic toxins (potassium, phosphate, sodium, hydrogen and urea-ammonium).

Our first foray into design of IJ catheters for dialysis was a fairly obvious idea, combining the implantation ease of a single body catheter with the improved hydraulic function of two separate tips. Thus, the Ash Split Cath™. Our next challenge was to diminish the incidence of catheter related infections (CRBSI) by an antiseptic and antithrombogenic catheter lock. Concentrated sodium citrate was successful in preventing CRBSI and catheter occlusion, but the FDA banned its use after a serious outcome resulting from misuse of the product. A product with low concentration of citrate and addition of antiseptics (Zuragen™) hit a brick wall within the FDA. We have continued with a project to obtain approval as a catheter lock to maintain patency of CVC for dialysis. This will be the first catheter lock solution to be approved for use in CVC for dialysis, of any kind.

As Winston Churchill said, "Success is never final, failure is not fatal, it is the courage to continue that counts." Whether it was your main goal or not, you have furthered the science of medicine by your development of a new device. Perhaps, you may have stimulated some other young physician or scientist to come up with a better idea.

CREDITS

A very special thanks for all your support:
Marianne Yeager Ash DVM, Emily Ash Morin MD and Sarah Ash Simpson LLD
Robert Truitt, MSE, MBA
Patti Truitt LLD
David Carr MSChe
Tom Sullivan BSEE

And thanks to so many others who assisted me and the numerous projects, in so many ways:

Jared Grantham	1
Willem Kolff	2, 4, 7, 9-12, 16, 92
Paul Malchesky	3
Vakhtang Tchantchaleishvili	3
Robert Truitt	2, 16, 19, 20, 26, 31, 40, 50, 68, 76
Stephen Jacobsen	4, 9, 10
Elizabeth Atkin-Thor	10
Robert Stephens	10
Charles Babbs	13
Les Geddes	13
Linda Wang	14
Joseph White	15
John Sherman	15, 39, 41
Patricia Truitt	20
Terry Echard	20
Kevin Sweeney	20

Carmine Durham	68,70
Paul Vajgrt	70
Bill Kennedy	75
Thomas Sullivan	82
Evan Koslow	82
Fokko Wieringa	89
Murray Sheldon	89
Emily Ash Morin	97
Sarah Ash Simpson	97
Marianne Ash	97
Dan Ulrich	104
Lawrence Weed	104
Marty Roberts	102

EPILOGUE

In this publication I have focused on one general goal of my life, improving the practice of dialysis. I suppose the real reason I wrote it was to convince myself that there was some unitary purpose or direction in my various research activities. Perhaps it was in response to those who claimed I had a "lack of focus" in my research projects. Well, maybe they're right. I do seem to have an inventor's penchant to focus on whatever problem seems to be the most urgent at the time. Apparent needs and frustrations lead an inventor almost immediately to think of solutions. If, fortunately or unfortunately, you soon think of a possible solution, you've hooked yourself. Then you've already got two reasons to do the project. In fact the only way I've found to free myself from fixation on a problem is to take my best idea about how to solve it, build a prototype, and test it to see whether it works or not.

The above twelve research projects were truly motivated by my feeling that we have a crisis in dialysis therapy, around the world. Besides being complicated, inconvenient, sometimes painful, and expensive, what else is wrong? It doesn't work very well, that's what. The mortality rate of ESRD patients on dialysis in the U.S. has improved somewhat in the past five years, but still hovers about 20% of patients per year. There is one way to improve outcomes of hemodialysis therapy, making it gentler and more effective in removal of middle-weight toxins, but this is practical only at home: increase the length and frequency of dialysis. So, this brings us back to my primary stimulus, finding ways to make dialysis simpler, safer and better suited for home use.

In this biography I have included projects that are related to hemodialysis only. For those readers who are not nephrologists, I didn't want them to have to do background reading on topics outside of hemodialysis, since that is com- plex enough. However, I have had a long and serious dedication to peritoneal dialysis, which is actually the mainstay of today's home dialysis therapy. While working with Dr. Kolff and others at the University of Utah in 1975, I saw first-hand that peritoneal dialysis worked, at least for patients with some residual kidney function. I learned how PD catheters were placed, and was introduced to the automated proportioning systems for in-center PD (Physio- Control and Drake-Willock). In the late 1970s, the first dialysis unit I managed in Lafayette, Indiana was an in-center peritoneal dialysis unit using proportioning machines by Physio-Control and Drake Willock. Very shortly after the description of CAPD by Moncrief and Popovich, we had patients at home per- forming the therapy (using glass bottles for each exchange). I formed a close relationship with Marty Roberts PhD, one of the originators of the Sorb column and its use in regenerating peritoneal dialysate.

I could write another biography regarding the projects I've performed to solve various problems in peritoneal dialysis (but don't worry I probably won't). Instead I'll just list them here, with the approximate years and the co- operating companies:

Year	Location	Project	Clinical Trials	FDA Approval	Outcome
1977	Bioengineeri-ng, Purdue	Column-Disc Catheter (LifeCath™), a catheter with Improved drainage and lack of migration.	Yes	Yes	Licensed to PhysioControl, successfully marketed, discontinued when company changed focus.
1981	Arnett Clinic	Y-Tec system for peritoneoscopic placement of PD catheters	No	Yes	System licensed to Medigroup, marketed widely, then acquired by Merit Medical.
1984	Ash Medical	Hydraulic Model of flow in peritoneum during PD, explaining outflow resistance and failure (with David Carr)	No	No	Analysis used by Baxter in design of HomeChoice software.
1997	Ash Medical	Continuous Flow Peritoneal Dialysis, animal study showing need for IP volume control for efficient clearance (with Dr. Elsa Janle Swain)	No	No	CFPD has been used more, especially in acute kidney failure in children Will combine perfectly with carbon block column.
1997	Ash Medical	T-Fluted PD Catheter (Advantage™), a PD catheter with external grooves (flutes) rather than side-holes, to improve peritoneal drainage., production problems.	Yes	Yes	Licensed to Medigroup. Improved outflow confirmed. Discontinued because placement procedure difficult,
2018	HemoCleanse Technology	Developed single-body slotted peritoneal catheter, for better drainage in PD and in HIPEC.	Soon	Not applied	Cooperation between ThermaSolutions and HemoCleanse Technology.
2018	HemoCleanse Technology, Purdue Bioengineering	Bioimpedance to measure IP volume during cycler PD therapy. Making the measurement system unobtrusive and comfortable.	Yes	No	In laboratory development, early clinical tests.

As you can see, my focus has been crystal clear, on anything that is re- motely related to improving home dialysis therapy.

Truthfully, my focus has wandered even more, from dialysis to other problems that vex me in my day-to-day practice of medicine. When I became frustrated with overweight patients I was seeing in clinic during Residency in

Internal Medicine, I invented the "Diet Plate" which would display how many calories were in a whole meal. It did receive a patent, but I never could find a company to market the thing. Same with the "Diet Fork," a utensil with a timer to slow the pace of eating for obese patients. I developed it due to frustration with overweight CKD patients in my Nephrology clinic. When joining the Arnett Clinic, a specialty clinic in Lafayette with about thirty-five doctors, I quickly learned that internal medicine specialists often provided full primary care to those patients who fit best in their specialty. That was especially true for me, since I was the first nephrologist ever hired by the clinic. Quickly I learned that patients with CKD and ESRD had numerous other complicated medical problems and I couldn't remember the main problems of each patient without a list. As soon as personal and portable computers (like the Apple II and HP 85) came on the market, I hired a bright young IT student from Purdue (Dan Ulrich) to implement the "Weed" system of problem-oriented patient care in a computer program (which ironically, Larry Weed never did). Eventually a solid but simple computer program evolved, which was then used in our dialysis unit and Nephrology practice for years. It became the first medical product sold by Ash Medical, and we called it first Total Recall™ and then SmartChart™.[124] We continued on the market the program until 2000. We didn't have the funds or market to allow us to adapt to the "Y2K" problem., In my own practice the computer had become indispensable by 2000.[125] As my clinic implemented the Epic and then finally the Cerner programs, I made sure that the detailed problem lists and other lists were electronically transferred, and worked with developers of these commercial programs to figure out how to use them in a manner in which the patient's problems were the prominent organizing feature of the data.

Besides medical problems, other frustrations also came from the affairs of living and owning a home. In 1975 Marianne and I purchased an 1870 farmhouse which became a major project in restoration for both of us. After we had the soffits and swale gutters replaced on the house, it pained me to see the drains repeatedly clog with leaves and damage the eaves. After years of trying to keep up with the problem, and trying various screen solutions, I learned that none of them worked. So, guess what? I started trying to invent new solutions, starting with ones that would work for twelve-inch wide, flat swale gutters and then adapting them to under-the-eave gutters. Marianne helped the project, often by telling me which ones would work and which wouldn't. Eventually we came to use a "slit separation" technique that my daughter Emily and I had tested for removing bubbles from a filtrate fluid in our lab. GutterShed™ remains on the market and has been licensed to a supportive family and company in West Virginia (see guttershed.com if you're re- ally curious and wish to see something new).

And there were a few other spurious directions, including studying dialysate iron for patients on hemodialysis[126] and running shoes with springs in them and an ice cream scoop with electric warming of the front edge, and even a CO2 powered rocket for personal protection. One happy result of many of these inventive efforts is that my whole family has a pretty good time sitting around the campfire or stove and talking about Dad's crazy inventions, especially my daughter Sarah.

On a more serious note, I don't think that I could have stayed in the practice of Nephrology and dialysis for over forty-seven years unless I had some hope that the future would be better for patients on dialysis. Now, with about 2 mil- lion people world-wide on some form of dialysis it is even more imperative to find truly new solutions and approaches to make dialysis simple, safe and suit- able for home. The recently implemented Advancing Americans Kidney Health (AAKH) executive order by President Trump and HHS is designed to increase utilization of home dialysis and transplantation. However, there is no significant funding for research into new and better technology and approaches. Rather than establishing penalties for physicians and programs that do not utilize home dialysis, wouldn't it be better to make more funding available for new improvements in dialysis? The recent KidneyX prizes by HHS and ASN have been helpful in highlighting the need for new ideas. But the total prize money is about $2 million. If one percent of the budget of NIH were directed towards improvements in ESRD therapy, that would be about $400 million. NIH might argue that prevention is a better goal than kidney replacement therapies. But how does prevention help patients who already have ESRD?

References

1 Ash SR. A lifelong quest to make home hemodialysis simple, safe, and effective: A review of outcomes of 12 major projects. Artif Organs. 2022 Jan;46(1):16-22.

2 Stephens RL, Jacobsen SC, Atkin-Thor E, Kolff W. Portable/wearable artificial kidney (WAK) - initial evaluation. Proc Eur Dial Transplant Assoc. 1976;12:511N518.

3 Dharnidharka SG, Kirkham R, Kolff WJ. Toward a wearable artificial kidney using ultrafiltrate as dialysate. Trans Am Soc Artif Intern Organs. 1973;19:92-7.

4 Kolff WJ, Jacobsen S, Stephen RL, Rose D. Towards a wearable artificial kidney. Kidney Int Suppl. 1976 Dec;(7):S300-4.

5 Stephen RL, Jacobsen SC, Kablitz C, Kolff WJ. Combined technological-clinical approach to wearable dialysis. Kidney Int Suppl. 1978 Jun;(8):S125-32.

6 Kolff WJ. Longitudinal perspectives on sorbents in uremia. Kidney Int Suppl. 1976 Dec;(7):S211-4.

7 Kolff W.J. (1979) The Future of Dialysis. In: Drukker W., Parsons F.M., Maher J.F. (eds) Replacement of Renal Function by Dialysis. Springer, Dordrecht. https://doi.org/10.1007/978-94-009-9327-3_42

8 Ash S. R.; Barile, R. G.; Thornhill, J. A.; Sherman, J. D.; Wang, N–H. L. In vivo evaluation of calcium-loaded zeolites and urease for urea removal in hemodialysis. Transactions - American Society for Artificial Internal Organs: April 1980 - Volume 26 - Issue 1 - p 111-115

9 Shihab-Eldeen AA, Peck GE, Ash SR, Kaufman G. Evaluation of the sorbent suspension reciprocating dialyser in the treatment of overdose of paracetamol and phenobarbitone. J Pharm Pharmacol. 1988;40(6):381N387. 10 KOLFF WJ, HIGGINS CC. Dialysis in the treatment of uremia: artificial kidney and peritoneal lavage. Trans Am Assoc Genitourin Surg. 1953;45:110-32.

11 Sherman JD. Synthetic zeolites and other microporous oxide molecular sieves. Proc Natl Acad Sci U S A. 1999 Mar 30;96(7):3471-8.

12 Ash SR, The Sorbent Suspension Reciprocating Dialyzer (SSRD); a Wearable Artificial Kidney that Almost Was. Artificial Organs 46 (2). 312-314, 2022

13 Gordon A, Better OS, Greenbaum MA, Marantz LB, Gral T, Maxwell MH. Clinical maintenance hemodialysis with a sorbent-based, low-volume dialysate regeneration system. Trans Am Soc Artif Intern Organs. 1971;17:253-8.

14 Blumenkrantz MJ, Gordon A, Roberts M, Lewin AJ, Pecker EA, Moran JK, Coburn JW, Maxwell MH. Applications of the Redy sorbent system to hemodialysis and peritoneal dialysis. Artif Organs. 1979 Aug;3(3):230-6.

15 Automatic priming, blood flow control, and rinsing during single access hemodialysis: the BioLogic-HD. Ash SR, Carr DJ, Baker K, Schultz T, Reynolds LO. Trans Am Soc Artif Intern Organs. 1985;31:499-503.

16 Badylak SF, Ash SR, Thornhill JA, Carr DJ. Doppler ultrasonic detection of particulate release during hemodialysis with cellulose hollow-fiber and sorbent suspension reciprocating dialyzers. Artif Organs. 1984 May;8(2):220-3.

17 Ash SR, Baker K, Blake DE, Carr DJ, Echard TG, Sweeney KD, Handt AE, Wimberly AL. Clinical trials of the BioLogic-HD. Automated single access, sorbent-based dialysis. ASAIO Trans. 1987 Jul-Sep;33(3):524- 31.

18 Higgins MR, Bettcher KB, Dossetor JB, Rice R, Mandin H, LeTourneau P. Cutting the costs of dialysis by using paid helpers. Can Med Assoc J. 1980;123(7):647-649.

19 MEDICARE Payments for Home Dialysis Much Higher Under Reasonable Charge Method, GAO/HRD publication 1989.

20 Kramer L, Kodras K. Detoxification as a treatment goal in hepatic failure. Liver Int. 2011 Sep;31 Suppl 3:1-4.

21 see ref 12.

22 Ash SR, BioLogic-HD™ and the Problem of being (way) too far ahead of the market, AO, V__ PP__.

23 Ash SR, Carr DJ, Blake DE, Rainier JB, Demetriou AA, Rozga J. Effect of sorbent-based dialytic therapy with the BioLogic-DT on an experimental model of hepatic failure. ASAIO J. 1993 Jul-Sep;39(3):M675-80.

24 Steczko J, Bax KC, Ash SR. Effect of hemodiabsorption and sorbent-based pheresis on amino acid levels in hepatic failure. Int J Artif Organs. 2000 Jun;23(6):375-88.

25 Ash SR, Blake DE, Carr DJ, Carter C, Howard T, Makowka L. Clinical effects of a sorbent suspension dialysis system in treatment of hepatic coma (the BioLogic-DT). Int J Artif Organs. 1992 Mar;15(3):151-61.

26 Ash SR, Caldwell CA, Singer GG, Lowell JA, Howard TK, Rustgi VK. Treatment of acetaminophen-induced hepatitis and fulminant hepatic failure with extracorporeal sorbent-based devices. Adv Ren Replace Ther. 2002 Jan;9(1):42-53.

27 Ash SR, Levy H, Akmal M, Mankus RA, Sutton JM, Emery DR, Scanlon JC, Blake DE, Carr DJ. Treatment of severe tricyclic antidepressant overdose with extracorporeal sorbent detoxification. Adv Ren Replace Ther. 2002 Jan;9(1):31-41.

28 Stange J, Mitzner SR, Risler T, Erley CM, Lauchart W, Goehl H, Klammt S, Peszynski P, Freytag J, Hickstein H, Löhr M, Liebe S, Schareck W, Hopt UT, Schmidt R. Molecular adsorbent recycling system (MARS): clinical results of a new membrane-based blood purification system for bioartificial liver support. Artif Organs. 1999 Apr;23(4):319-30.

29 Patzer JF 2nd, Bane SE. Bound solute dialysis. ASAIO J. 2003 May-Jun;49(3):271-81.

30 Stange J, Mitzner SR, Risler T, Erley CM, Lauchart W, Goehl H, Klammt S, Peszynski P, Freytag J, Hickstein H, Löhr M, Liebe S, Schareck W, Hopt UT, Schmidt R. Molecular adsorbent recycling system (MARS): clinical results of a new membrane-based blood purification system for bioartificial liver support. Artif Organs. 1999 Apr;23(4):319-30.

31 Mitzner SR, Stange J, Klammt S, Peszynski P, Schmidt R, Nöldge-Schomburg G. Extracorporeal detoxification using the molecular adsorbent recirculating system for critically ill patients with liver failure. J Am Soc Nephrol. 2001 Feb;12 Suppl 17:S75-82.

32 Stange J, Hassanein TI, Mehta R, Mitzner SR, Bartlett RH. The molecular adsorbents recycling system as a liver support system based on albumin dialysis: a summary of preclinical investigations, prospective, randomized, controlled clinical trial, and clinical experience from 19 centers. Artif Organs. 2002 Feb;26(2):103-10.

33 Kramer L, Gendo A, Madl C, Ferrara I, Funk G, Schenk P, Sunder-Plassmann G, Hörl WH. Biocompatibility of a cuprophane charcoal-based detoxification device in cirrhotic patients with hepatic encephalopathy. Am J Kidney Dis. 2000 Dec;36(6):1193-200.

34 Steczko J, Ash SR, Blake DE, Carr DJ, Bosley RH. Cytokines and endotoxin removal by sorbents and its application in push-pull sorbent-based pheresis: the BioLogic-DTPF System. Artif Organs. 1999 Apr;23(4):310-8

35 Steinhart CR, Ash SR, Gingrich C, Sapir D, Keeling GN, Yatvin MB. Effect of whole-body hyperthermia on AIDS patients with Kaposi's sarcoma: a pilot study. J Acquir Immune Defic Syndr Hum Retrovirol. 1996 Mar 1;11(3):271-81.

36 Ash SR, Steinhart CR, Curfman MF, Gingrich CH, Sapir DA, Ash EL, Fausset JM, Yatvin MB. Extracorporeal whole body hyperthermia treatments for HIV infection and AIDS. ASAIO J. 1997 Sep-Oct;43(5):M830-8.

37 Zwischenberger JB, Vertrees RA, Bedell EA, McQuitty CK, Chernin JM, Woodson LC. Percutaneous ven-ovenous perfusion-induced systemic hyperthermia for lung cancer: a phase I safety study. Ann Thorac Surg. 2004 Jun;77(6):1916-24; discussion 1925.

38 Lockridge RS Jr, Moran J. Short daily hemodialysis and nocturnal hemodialysis at home: practical considerations. Semin Dial. 2008 Jan-Feb;21(1):49-53.

39 Ash SR. BioLogic-HD and the problem of being (way) too far ahead of the market. Artif Organs. 2022 Feb 9 (e-pub).

40 Ash SR. The Allient dialysis system. Semin Dial. 2004 Mar-Apr;17(2):164-6.

41 Roberts M, Lee DBN, Ash SR, Loke G and Ku G. Sorbent Dialysis and the Wearable Artificial Kidney.. In: Ing TS, Rahman MA, Kjellstrand CM (eds). Dialysis: History, Development and Promise. New Jersey. World Scientific, 2012 561-568.

42 Ash SR. Sorbents in treatment of uremia: a short history and a great future. Semin Dial. 2009 Nov-Dec;22(6):615-22.

43 Rosenbaum BP, Ash SR, Wong RJ, Thompson RP, Carr DJ. Prediction of hemodialysis sorbent cartridge urea nitrogen capacity and sodium release from in vitro tests. Hemodial Int. 2008 Apr;12(2):244-53

44 AAMI TIR77: Sorbent-based regenerative hemodialysis systems. AAMI, Arlington, VA, 2018

45 Shu F, Parks R, Maholtz J, Ash S, Antaki JF. Multimodal flow visualization and optimization of pneumatic blood pump for sorbent hemodialysis system. Artif Organs. 2009 Apr;33(4):334-45

46 McGill RL, Bakos JR, Ko T, Sandroni SE, Marcus RJ. Sorbent hemodialysis: clinical experience with new sorbent cartridges and hemodialyzers. ASAIO J. 2008 Nov-Dec;54(6):618-21.

47 Ash SR. A lifelong quest to make home hemodialysis simple, safe, and effective: A review of outcomes of 12 major projects. Artif Organs. 2022 Jan;46(1):16-22.

48 Ash SR. A lifelong quest to make home hemodialysis simple, safe, and effective: A review of outcomes of 12 major projects. Artif Organs. 2022 Jan;46(1):16-22..

49 see ref 12

50 Sinclair A, Babbs CF, Griffin DD, Ash SR. Roux-Y intestinal bypass for administration of sorbents in uremia. Kidney Int Suppl. 1978 Jun;(8):S153-9.

51 Bem, David S.; Sherman, John D.; Ash, Stephen R.; Marte, Julio C.; Willis, Richard R.; Braun, Richard; Muldoon, Brian S.. ammonium REMOVAL WITH A NOVEL ZIRCONIUM SILICATE. ASAIO Journal: March-April 2001 - Volume 47 - Issue 2 - p 151. (abstract)

52 Ash, SR. Allient™ Hemodialysis Machine; Sorbent-Based, Single-Needle Sorbent Dialysis Reborn. Artificial Organs, 46(5), 972-976, 2022

53 Ash, SR. Cation Exchangers as Oral Sorbents for Ammonium and Potassium: PSS, ZP and ZS (Zirconium Silicate). ASAIO Innovation Conference, 2007 (abstract).

54 Ash SR, Singh B, Lavin PT, Stavros F, Rasmussen HS. A phase 2 study on the treatment of hyperkalemia in patients with chronic kidney disease suggests that the selective potassium trap, SZC, is safe and efficient. Kidney Int. 2015 Aug;88(2):404-11.

55 Metcalfe-Gibson A, Ing TS, Kuiper JJ, Richards P, Ward EE, Wrong OM. In vivo dialysis of faeces as a method of stool analysis. II. The influence of diet. Clin Sci. 1967 Aug;33(1):89-100.

56 Wilson DR, Ing TS, Metcalfe-Gibson A, Wrong OM. The chemical composition of faeces in uraemia, as revealed by in-vivo faecal dialysis. Clin Sci. 1968 Oct;35(2):197-209.

57 Roger SD, Spinowitz BS, Lerma EV, Singh B, Packham DK, Al-Shurbaji A, Kosiborod M. Efficacy and Safety of Sodium SZC for Treatment of Hyperkalemia: An 11-Month Open-Label Extension of HARMO- NIZE. Am J Nephrol. 2019;50(6):473-480..

58 Ash SR, Singh B, Lavin PT, Stavros F, Rasmussen HS. "Safety and Efficacy of SZC, a Novel Selective Cation Trap, for Treatment of Hyperkalemia in CKD Patients." Presentation at American Society of Nephrol- ogy, Atlanta, GA, November 8, 2013.

59 Roger SD, Spinowitz BS, Lerma EV, Fishbane S, Ash SR, Martins JG, Quinn CM, Packham DK. Sodium SZC increases serum bicarbonate concentrations among patients with hyperkalaemia: exploratory analyses from three randomized, multi-dose, placebo-controlled trials. Nephrol Dial Transplant. 2020 Jun 26:gfaa158.

60 Kosiborod M, Rasmussen HS, Lavin P, Qunibi WY, Spinowitz B, Packham D, Roger SD, Yang A, Lerma E, Singh B. Effect of sodium SZC on potassium lowering for 28 days among outpatients with hyperkalemia: the HARMONIZE randomized clinical trial. JAMA. 2014 Dec 3;312(21):2223-33.

61 Packham DK, Rasmussen HS, Lavin PT, El-Shahawy MA, Roger SD, Block G, Qunibi W, Pergola P, Singh B. Sodium SZC in hyperkalemia. N Engl J Med. 2015 Jan 15;372(3):222-31.

62 Fishbane S, Ford M, Fukagawa M, McCafferty K, Rastogi A, Spinowitz B, Staroselskiy K, Vishnevskiy K, Lisovskaja V, Al-Shurbaji A, Guzman N, Bhandari S. A Phase 3b, Randomized, Double-Blind, Placebo-Controlled Study of Sodium SZC for Reducing the Incidence of Predialysis Hyperkalemia. J Am Soc Nephrol. 2019 Sep;30(9):1723-1733.

63 Fishbane S, Ford M, Fukagawa M, McCafferty K, Rastogi A, Spinowitz B, Staroselskiy K, Vishnevskiy K, Lisovskaja V, Al-Shurbaji A, Guzman N, Bhandari S. A Phase 3b, Randomized, Double-Blind, Placebo-Controlled Study of Sodium SZC for Reducing the Incidence of Predialysis Hyperkalemia. J Am Soc Nephrol. 2019 Sep;30(9):1723-1733.

64 Stephen Richard Ash, David John Carr. Oral sorbent for removing toxins of kidney failure combining anion and cation exchangers. US Patent Number US10668098B2. Granted 2020-06-02.

65 Sinclair A, Griffin DD, Voreis JD, Ash SR. Sorbent binding of urea and creatinine in a Roux-Y intestinal segment. Clin Nephrol. 1979 Feb;11(2):97-104..

66 Shaldon S: Percutaneous vessel catheterization for hemodialysis. ASAIO J 40:17-19, 1994

67 Uldall PR, Joy C, Merchant N. Further experience with a double-lumen subclavian cannula for hemodialysis. Trans Am Soc Artif Intern Organs. 1982;28:71-5.

68 Mahurkar SD: The fluid mechanics of hemodialysis catheters. Trans Am Soc Artif Intern Organs 31:124- 130, 1985.

69 Ash SR. The evolution and function of central venous catheters for dialysis. Seminars in Dialysis 14:416- 424, 2002.

70 Tesio F, De Baz H, Panarello G, Calianno G, Quaia P, Raimondi A, Schinella D. Double catheterization of the internal jugular vein for hemodialysis: indications, techniques, and clinical results. Artif Organs. 1994 Apr;18(4):301-4.

71 Canaud B, Leray-Moragues H, Kerkeni N, Bosc JY, Martin K. Effective flow performances and dialysis doses delivered with permanent catheters: a 24-month comparative study of permanent catheters versus ar- terio-venous vascular accesses. Nephrol Dial Transplant. 2002 Jul;17(7):1286-92.

72 Ash SR. Fluid mechanics and clinical success of central venous catheters for dialysis--answers to simple but persisting problems. Semin Dial. 2007 May-Jun;20(3):237-56.

73 Ash SR, Mankus RA, Sutton JM, Spray M. The Ash Split Cath as long-term IJ access: hydraulic performance and longevity. J Vascular Access 3:3-9, 2002.

74 Agarwal AK, Ash SR; Principal Investigators of the CentrosFLO Trial. Maintenance of blood flow rate on dialysis with self-centering CentrosFLO catheter: A multicenter prospective study. Hemodial Int. 2016 Oct;20(4):501-509.

75 To a Mouse by Robert Burns - Scottish Poetry Library

76 Ash SR. The "Ash Split-Cath"; The Best Inventions are Simple. Artif Organs V46 (7)

77 Ash SR, BioLogic-HD™ and the Problem of being (way) too far ahead of the market, Artif Organs, V46 (3).

78 Twardowski ZJ, Reams G, Prowant BF, Moore HL, Van Stone JC. Air-bubble method of locking central-vein catheters for prevention of hub colonization: a pilot study. Hemodial Int. 2003 Oct 1;7(4):320-5.

79 Ash SR, Mankus RA, Sutton JM, Criswell RE, Crull CC, Velasquez KA, Smeltzer BD, Ing TS. Concentrated Sodium Citrate (23%) for Catheter Lock. Hemodial Int. 2000 Jan;4(1):22-31.

80 Polaschegg HD. Loss of catheter locking solution caused by fluid density. ASAIO J. 2005 May-Jun;51(3):230-5.

81 https://www.infectioncontroltoday.com/view/warning-about-tricitrasol

82 Silva J, Antunes J, Carvalho T, Ponce P. Efficacy of preventing hemodialysis catheter infections with citrate lock. Hemodial Int. 2012 Oct;16(4):545-52.

83 Allon M. Prophylaxis against dialysis catheter-related bacteremia: a glimmer of hope. Am J Kidney Dis. 2008 Feb;51(2):165-8.

84 Fisher M, Golestaneh L, Allon M, Abreo K, Mokrzycki MH. Prevention of Bloodstream Infections in Patients Undergoing Hemodialysis. Clin J Am Soc Nephrol. 2020 Jan 7;15(1):132-151.

85 Ash SR, Mankus RA, Sutton JM, Criswell RE, Crull CC, Velasquez KA, Smeltzer BD, Ing TS. Concentrated Sodium Citrate (23%) for Catheter Lock. Hemodial Int. 2000 Jan;4(1):22-31.

86 Steczko J, Ash SR, Nivens DE, Brewer L, Winger RK. Microbial inactivation properties of a new antimicrobial/antithrombotic catheter lock solution (citrate/methylene blue/parabens). Nephrol Dial Transplant. 2009 Jun;24(6):1937-45.

87 Sauer K, Steczko J, Ash SR. Effect of a solution containing citrate/methylene blue/parabens on Staphylococcus Aureus bacteria and biofilm and comparison with various heparin solutions. J Antimicrob Chemother. 2009 May; 63(5):937-45.

88 Quittnat Pelletier F, Joarder M, Poutanen SM, Lok CE. Evaluating Approaches for the Diagnosis of Hemodialysis Catheter-Related Bloodstream Infections. Clin J Am Soc Nephrol. 2016 May 6;11(5):847-54..

89 Maki DG, Ash SR, Winger RK, Lavin P; for the AZEPTIC Trial Investigators. A novel antimicrobial and antithrombotic lock solution for hemodialysis catheters: A multi-center, controlled, randomized trial. Crit Care Med 2011 Vol. 39, No. 4, 613-620.

90 Ash SR. Zuragen™ Antiseptic Catheter Lock: A Bridge Too Far? Art Organs 46 (9), pending publication.

91 Maki DG, Ash SR, Winger RK, Lavin P; for the AZEPTIC Trial Investigators. A novel antimicrobial and antithrombotic lock solution for hemodialysis catheters: A multi-center, controlled, randomized trial. Crit Care Med 2011 Vol. 39, No. 4, 613-620.

92 Steczko J, Ash SR, Brewer L, Guillem A. In vitro and in vivo evaluation of efficacy of citrate/methylene blue/parabens/IPA solution as a skin disinfectant. J Infect. 2010 Jan;60(1):36-43.

93 Kampf G. Acquired resistance to chlorhexidine: is it time to establish an antiseptic stewardship' initiative? J Hosp Infect 2016; 94:213–227.

94 Williamson DA, Carter GP, and Howden BP. Current and emerging topical antibacterials and antiseptics: agents, action, and resistance patterns. Clin Microbiol Rev 2017;30 827–860.

95 Addetia A, Greninger AL, Adler A, et al. A novel, widespread qaca allele results in reduced chlorhexidine susceptibility in Staphylococcus epidermidis. Antimicrob Agents Chemother 2019;63(6): pii: e02607-18.

96 FDA drug safety podcast: FDA warns about rare but serious allergic reactions with the skin antiseptic chlorhexidine gluconate. Food and Drug Administration website. https://www.fda.gov/Drugs/DrugSafety/DrugSafetyPodcasts/ucm540654.htm. Published 2017. Accessed August 12, 2019.

97 ZuraGard | Zurex Pharma.

98 Crnich CJ, Pop-Vicas AE, Hedberg TG, Perl TM. Efficacy and safety of a novel antimicrobial preoperative skin preparation. Infect Control Hosp Epidemiol. 2019 Oct;40(10):1157-1163.

99 Edmiston CE, Lavin P, Spencer M, Borlaug G, Seabrook GR, Leaper D. Antiseptic efficacy of an innovative perioperative surgical skin preparation: A confirmatory FDA phase 3 analysis. Infect Control Hosp Epidemiol. 2020 Jun;41(6):653-659..

100 Ascribed to numerous people, but first appeared in print in Danish in 1948, It's Difficult to Make Predictions, Especially About the Future – Quote Investigator

101 Ash SR, Mankus RA, Sutton JM, Criswell RE, Crull CC, Velasquez KA, Smeltzer BD, Ing TS. Concentrated Sodium Citrate (23%) for Catheter Lock. Hemodial Int. 2000 Jan;4(1):22-31.

102 Ash SR, Concentrated Sodium Citrate Catheter Lock; "The best laid schemes o' mice an' men…" Artificial Organs 46 (8), 1701-1704, 2022.

103 Fisher M, Golestaneh L, Allon M, Abreo K, Mokrzycki MH. Prevention of Bloodstream Infections in Patients Undergoing Hemodialysis. Clin J Am Soc Nephrol. 2020 Jan 7;15(1):132-151.

104 Moran JE, Ash SR, ASDIN Clinical Practice Committee. Locking solutions for hemodialysis catheters; heparin and citrate--a position paper by ASDIN. Semin Dial. 2008 Sep-Oct; 21(5):490-2.

105 Huang HM, Jiang X, Meng LB, Di CY, Guo P, Qiu Y, Dai YL, Lv XQ, Shi CJ. Reducing catheter-associated complications using 4% sodium citrate versus sodium heparin as a catheter lock solution. J Int Med Res. 2019 Sep;47(9):4204-4214.

106 Yon CK, Low CL. Sodium citrate 4% versus heparin as a lock solution in hemodialysis patients with central venous catheters. Am J Health Syst Pharm. 2013 Jan 15;70(2):131-6.

107 Moran J, Sun S, Khababa I, Pedan A, Doss S, Schiller B. A randomized trial comparing gentamicin/citrate and heparin locks for central venous catheters in maintenance hemodialysis patients. Am J Kidney Dis. 2012 Jan;59(1):102-7.

108 Polaschegg HD. Loss of catheter locking solution caused by fluid density. ASAIO J. 2005 May-Jun;51(3):230-5.

109 Maki DG, Ash SR, Winger RK, Lavin P; AZEPTIC Trial Investigators. A novel antimicrobial and antithrombotic lock solution for hemodialysis catheters: a multi-center, cont™lled, randomized trial. Crit Care Med. 2011 Apr;39(4):613-20.

110 Ash SR, Zuragen™®; A Bridge Too Far? Artificial Organs V46 (9), pp__ 2021

111 See ref 52.

112 Stephen Richard Ash, David John Carr. Oral sorbent for removing toxins of kidney failure combining anion and cation exchangers. US Patent Number US10668098B2. Granted 2020-06-02.

113 Ash SR. Zirconium cyclosilicate: an oral sorbent for potassium, four decades in the making. Artificial Organs 46(6), 1192-1197, 2022

114 Kosiborod M, Rasmussen HS, Lavin P, Qunibi WY, Spinowitz B, Packham D, Roger SD, Yang A, Lerma E, Singh B. Effect of sodium zirconium cyclosilicate on potassium lowering for 28 days among outpatients with hyperkalemia: the HARMONIZE randomized clinical trial. JAMA. 2014 Dec 3;312(21):2223-33.

115 Packham DK, Rasmussen HS, Lavin PT, El-Shahawy MA, Roger SD, Block G, Qunibi W, Pergola P, Singh B. Sodium zirconium cyclosilicate in hyperkalemia. N Engl J Med. 2015 Jan 15;372(3):222-31.

116 Fishbane S, Ford M, Fukagawa M, McCafferty K, Rastogi A, Spinowitz B, Staroselskiy K, Vishnevskiy K, Lisovskaja V, Al-Shurbaji A, Guzman N, Bhandari S. A Phase 3b, Randomized, Double-Blind, Placebo-Controlled Study of Sodium Zirconium Cyclosilicate for Reducing the Incidence of Predialysis Hyper-kalemia. J Am Soc Nephrol. 2019 Sep;30(9):1723-1733.

117 Stephen Ash, David Carr, Tom Sullivan. Carbon block/filtration bed/conical reactor with fluidized bed system allowing small sorbent particles to regenerate fluid during extracorporeal blood treatment. U.S. Patent number: 10702797 issued July 7, 2020.

118 Large Scale Production of Extruded Carbon Block Filter Cartridges—A Case Study Posted: Monday, May 15th, 2000 in 2000, Carbon Filtration, Evan E. Koslow, May, Spotlight, Writer

119 Gura V, Macy AS, Beizai M, Ezon C, Golper TA. Technical breakthroughs in the wearable artificial kidney (WAK). Clin J Am Soc Nephrol. 2009 Sep;4(9):1441-8.

120 Archdeacon P, Shaffer RN, Winkelmayer WC, Falk RJ, Roy-Chaudhury P. Fostering innovation, advancing patient safety: the kidney health initiative. Clin J Am Soc Nephrol. 2013 Sep; 8(9):1609-17.

121 Wieringa FP, Sheldon M. The Kidney Health Initiative innovation roadmap for renal replacement therapies: Building the yellow brick road, while updating the map. Artif Organs. 2020 Feb; 44(2):111-122.

122 Ash SR, Groth T, Wieringa FP. Summary of the 2020 IFAO-ASAIO Session on Implantable Artificial Kidney. ASAIO J. 2020 Aug 6.

123 Ash SR. Artificial Organs: a new chapter in medical history. ASAIO J 2006 Nov-Dec; 52(6):e3-9.

124 Ash SR. Mertz SL, and Ulrich DK. The computerized notation system: a portable, self-contained system for entry of physicians' and nurses' notes. Proc SCAMC, p. 129-135, 1981, and J of Clinical Engineering, 8:2:147-155, April/June 1983.

125 Ash SR. Computer-based charting (Part I). Physicians & Computers 14(7):24-35, 1997. (Part II). Physicians & Computers 14(8):16-35, 1997.

126 Stephen Ash US patent US20050148663A1. Method for iron delivery to a patient by transfer from dialysate. Published 2005-07-07.